Good Clinical P
Standard Operating Pro
Clinical Researchers

Edited by

Josef Kolman

MPRC – Medical Pharmaceutical Research Center Ltd, Vienna, Austria

Paul Meng

PMC – Dr Paul Meng Consultant, Vienna, Austria

and

Graeme Scott

Professional Services in Clinical Research, Edinburgh, Scotland

JOHN WILEY & SONS

Chichester • New York • Weinheim • Brisbane • Singapore • Toronto

Other Wiley Editorial Offices

John Wiley & Sons, Inc., 605 Third Avenue,
New York, NY 10158-0012, USA

WILEY-VCH Verlag GmbH, Pappelallee 3,
D-69469 Weinheim, Germany

Jacaranda Wiley Ltd, 33 Park Road, Milton,
Queensland 4064, Australia

John Wiley & Sons (Asia) Pte Ltd, 2 Clementi Loop #02-01,
Jin Xing Distripark, Singapore 129809

John Wiley & Sons (Canada) Ltd, 22 Worcester Road,
Rexdale, Ontario M9W 1L1, Canada

Library of Congress Cataloging-in-Publication Data

Good clinical practice : standard operating procedures for clinical
  researchers / edited by Josef Kolman, Paul Meng and Graeme Scott.
      p. cm.
    Includes bibliographical references and index.
    ISBN 0-471-96936-2 (paper : alk. paper)
    1. Clinical trials—Standards. I. Kolman, Josef. II. Meng,
Paul. III. Scott, Graeme.
    [DNLM: 1. Clinical Trials—standards. 2. Research Design—
standards.   QV 771 G6465 1998]
    R853.C55G66 1998
    610'.72—dc21   97–41919
                                                                      CIP

British Library Cataloguing in Publication Data

A catalogue record for this book is available from the British Library

ISBN 0-471-96936-2

Typeset in 10/12pt Times by Mayhew Typesetting, Rhayader, Powys

This book is printed on acid-free paper responsibly manufactured from sustainable forestry,
in which at least two trees are planted for each one used for paper production.

Printed and bound by Antony Rowe Ltd, Eastbourne

Contents

Contributors

Helen Curley
Pharmakopius (Europe) Ltd, Alexander House, Gatehampton Road, Goring on Thames, Reading RG8 0EN, UK

Josef Kolman
MPRC – Medical Pharmaceutical Research Center Ltd, Hernalser Haupstrasse 24/16, A-1170 Vienna, Austria

Penny Maguire
Institute of Cardiovascular Research, Worsley Building, University of Leeds, Leeds LS2 9JT, UK

Paul Meng
PMC – Dr Paul Meng Consultant, Hernalser Haupstrasse 24/16, A-1170 Vienna, Austria

Adolf Pohl
Heidelweg 5, A-1140 Vienna, Austria

Graeme Scott
Professional Services in Clinical Research, One Buckstane Park, Edinburgh EH10 6PA, Scotland

Mary Thompson
Research Sister, Rotherham Hospital Trust, Moorgate Road, Rotherham, South Yorkshire S60 2UD, UK

Foreword

If anything can go wrong, it will.
Murphy's Law

Standard Operating Procedures (SOPs) have become the normal way by which Sponsor pharmaceutical and medical device companies document the processes they adopt for the initiation, conduct and reporting of clinical trials, i.e. attempt to minimise the effects of Murphy's Law. Adoption of SOPs has progressed in parallel with the evolution of GCP (see Introduction) and the various GCP guidelines require Sponsors to maintain a sufficiently comprehensive and up-to-date set of SOPs.

The SOP concept was not universally welcomed within Sponsor companies but, with time, a number of benefits have been clearly demonstrated:

1. It provides a written record of the process
2. Processes used by several individuals are applied (more) consistently
3. Team members' confidence is increased and performance is enhanced
4. It helps with the training of new staff
5. Reduces supervisory time/effort.

One of the key objectives of clinical trials is the generation of quality data. Quality has to be built into a clinical study from the outset, i.e. starting at the study design stage and continuing through all subsequent stages. The contribution of the Investigator and all members of the study site team participating and supporting the trial is clearly critical to the quality of the data generated. In view of this and the benefits that SOPs can produce, Investigators should consider introducing SOPs for those processes that are relevant to the type of clinical trial work carried out at their study site.

This book provides a comprehensive 'bank' of SOPs to enable Investigators to generate a set which is appropriate for their use with the minimum of effort. This can be achieved by customising those selected, e.g. to reflect the specific organisation of the site. If greater specificity is desired, the degree of customisation can be increased. The benefit of this publication is that the basic SOP structures are ready made, minimising the effort needed to construct a portfolio of relevant SOPs.

This initiative will be useful to anyone that is interested in adopting SOPs at their study site.

Tom Gallacher
Head, Clinical SOPs
SmithKline Beecham Pharmaceuticals

Acknowledgements

The editors would like to acknowledge both the significant contribution made by Pamela Waltl, whose hard work, organisation and language skills made the original manuscript for this book possible, and the expert and patient assistance of Helen Green with the production of drafts of this text.

Introduction

These Standard Operating Procedures (SOPs) for Investigators have been written for the use of doctors and their staff performing clinical research in hospitals and general practice.

Since the mid-1980s there have been great changes in the way clinical research is performed, with the almost universal introduction of Good Clinical Practice (GCP) in one form or another. Any doctor performing any form of clinical research needs to be aware of the relevant GCP Guidelines.

These SOPs have been written to make your job easier in performing clinical research. If you work according to the written procedures with the accompanying checklists, then not only will you be working according to the GCP Guidelines, you will also be producing high quality clinical research.

The International Conference on Harmonisation of Technical Requirements for the Registration of Pharmaceuticals for Human Use (ICH) is in the process of introducing sets of guidelines for the development and production of drugs to enable research to be done cost effectively, with less duplication of effort and reduction in exposure of animals and humans. The ICH harmonised tripartite guideline for Good Clinical Practice[1] reached step four of the ICH process on 1st May 1996 and came into operation for clinical trials commencing after 17th January 1997. They provide what is effectively a single standard for the conduct of clinical trials anywhere in the world. Adherence to the guidelines will make the data generated at your study site useful for regulatory submissions in European countries, North America, Japan and all other world markets.

Study sites already adhering to European GCP Guidelines will find the impact of ICH GCP on their working procedures small; it is Sponsors and Independent Ethics Committees for whom the guidelines are likely to have more effect. As a 'study site', the work you and your staff do on behalf of the pharmaceutical industry is probably done, at least partly, on a commercial basis: the money earned from such clinical research can be important in generating funds for other research or patient care. The ability to conduct trials to a consistently high standard is increasingly becoming one of the most important deciding factors in the placing of clinical trials at study sites. Site SOPs are an essential tool in ensuring consistent attainment of high standards by all relevant staff. Checklists help ensure that all requirements of GCP, whether it be ICH or European, are met, but in an increasingly commercial and competitive market place, good SOPs and close adherence to them can be the difference between getting or losing a new contract.

In the first section of this text, there is a brief description of the history and development of clinical research and GCP, then an explanation of what Standard Operating Procedures are and how they should work, and then the main body of the text comprising the SOPs and checklists.

CLINICAL RESEARCH

The development of a new drug is a long and complicated business. The role of the doctor performing clinical research (i.e. the Investigator) is a critical one. The aim of this summary is to give you a background knowledge of drug development so that you can better appreciate the importance of your role in producing high quality results in ethical clinical research.

Most of the drugs which are used in medicine today have, after their initial discovery, undergone a range of laboratory tests using cell cultures, isolated tissues and animals.

If a drug shows clinical potential, it may be used in humans only after successful completion of pre-clinical toxicity tests on different animal species (these are conducted according to another set of regulations known as Good Laboratory Practice – GLP).

For every 50,000 or so substances which are synthesised in the laboratory, approximately five will reach the stage of tests in humans – only one of these will actually be safe and effective enough to be marketed.

PHASES OF A CLINICAL TRIAL

After much of the laboratory testing is completed, the first use of the drug in humans can take place. The tests on humans can be classified into four phases (see Table 1). Although there are no strict definitions or internationally recognised norms for the phases, the following is generally accepted:

Phase I

Phase I trials are normally done on healthy volunteers, usually in special hospital units equipped for performing these trials. Studies on the drug's absorption, distribution, metabolism and excretion (pharmacokinetics) are done – as few as 10 to 20 volunteers may take part in a Phase I trial.

Phase II

Phase II trials are generally the first trials in patients, conducted mainly to give an idea of efficacy, to identify the optimal dose and to provide the first indications on safety in patients. Differences in the pharmacokinetics between healthy volunteers and patients are also assessed. Up to a few hundred patients are involved in this phase and it is not uncommon for the studies to be uncontrolled or only loosely controlled.

Phase III

Phase III trials are the main assessment of safety and efficacy of a drug. Many more patients are treated in Phase III trials; it can be as many as several thousand. There are several different types of trial design and these will be mentioned later but Phase III trials are generally rigorously controlled studies; most regulatory authorities insist on this phase being a randomised, comparative study. The results of Phase III trials are usually those that are pivotal in obtaining approval of the authorities for marketing of the drug. A product may require anything from 10 to 80 different trials involving up to 3000 patients or more for the registration.

Phase IV

Phase IV trials are those performed after obtaining a licence to market the drug. Here, in contrast to Phases II and III, problems associated with long term use of the drug or rare adverse effects can be detected. New dosages and indications may also be tested in Phase IV trials.

From discovery to registration may typically take from 10 to 12 years and involves huge costs: approximately 100 million pounds sterling or more (approximately 250 million Deutschmarks).

Table 1. Phases of clinical trials

Phase	Population	Typical Numbers Involved per Protocol	Comments
I	Healthy volunteers	10–20	First use in humans, pharmacokinetics
II	Patients	100–200	Assess efficacy, optimal dose, first indications on safety
III	Patients	300–several thousand	Efficacy and safety, comparison against standard, pivotal data for registration
IV	Patients	Variable	Long term efficacy and safety, assessment of rare adverse events

CLINICAL TRIAL DESIGN

There are several different types of design of clinical trial with varying degrees of complexity. Only a brief overview can be given here – you are advised to consult standard texts for further information.[2] If you are invited to work in a trial and you are not familiar with any aspect of the trial design, the Sponsor's medical adviser or Monitor should take the time to explain the study to you. It is vital that you understand not only the clinical side to the trial but also the theory of clinical research.

Earlier, two of the most important terms in clinical trial design were mentioned: *randomised* and *comparative*.

The purpose of randomisation is to avoid bias. It means the random allocation of patients to one of the study treatments. This means that when a patient comes to your clinic and agrees to take part in a randomised trial, neither you nor the patient know to which treatment group they will be allocated. Be sure that you know exactly what the randomisation procedure is for each study. It should be stated in the study protocol. A common method is for the study medication to be packed and numbered according to a separate randomisation list. When a patient is to be enrolled in the study they are given the next available numbered packet.

Stratification is a more sophisticated form of randomisation and is used, for example, when a different treatment response might be expected from different groups of patients; examples are between renally impaired patients and those with normal kidney function or between male and female patients. It then ensures that roughly equal numbers of, in the latter case, men and women will be allocated to each treatment group, removing the possibility that, by chance, there is an uneven distribution of the sexes between groups, making comparison of the results flawed.

Clinical research is constantly developing to meet new needs, and it may be that in addition to the well known randomised, controlled study you may be asked to assess quality of life or make some kind of economic assessment of the illness or the treatment.

Some types of trial design are listed in Figure 1.

Figure 1. Trial design

Comparative or controlled studies:
- reference drug
- no treatment
- placebo

Open/Blind trials
- Open
- Single blind
- Double blind
- Double dummy

Parallel group design
Matched pairs

Crossover studies (run-in and wash-out periods)
Factorial design (e.g. for comparing combinations of treatment)

Sequential

Quality of life studies
Cost–benefit studies

HISTORY AND DEVELOPMENT OF GCP

One of the reasons that GCP was introduced and accepted was because of concern *about drug safety*. In particular there was public anxiety among regulators about the quality and reliability of some of the research data submitted to the regulatory authorities. Fraudulent data could jeopardise patient safety or could cause the rejection of an application for a new drug – and could cost the pharmaceutical company millions of pounds. Fraudulent data have usually emphasised the efficacy and underplayed the toxicity of a drug.

Examples of fraudulence range from modification of data to deliberate fabrication of results. In more than one case the data from one patient has been used in two different studies; one gynaecologist fabricated data for over 900 patients! The data may also be modified to improve acceptability, or to improve chances of publication: for example reporting that a pre-treatment radiograph is worse than it actually is, so that the treatment appears better.

There have also been flagrant, but non-deliberate, violations of research norms and regulations: one Investigator reported normal liver tests shortly before the patient died of hepatic failure.[3]

The European Guidelines for Good Clinical Practice for Trials on Medicinal Products in the European Community[4] were introduced in 1991, but the idea of GCP originated and was developed in the USA. In the USA there is a much longer history of drug regulation, starting in 1813 with a smallpox Vaccine Act.[5] In addition to this there are cultural differences, with a much more questioning and less trusting attitude which made the introduction of GCP easier than in Europe.

In the early 1960s the thalidomide disaster caused a tightening of government regulations both in Europe and the USA, but it was in 1977 that the Food and Drug Administration (FDA) introduced a set of proposals for Investigators and Sponsors of clinical trials.

There was, however, no internationally recognised standard and this caused problems with the recognition of data from foreign studies for the registration of new drugs in the USA. This meant that studies often had to be repeated in the USA, to meet FDA standards.

Between 1986 and 1990 individual European countries did start to introduce guidelines along the lines of the US regulations and in 1990 an EC Working Party published the EC GCP Guidelines which have been introduced into the national laws of several individual member states – Ireland, France, Germany and Spain have all legislated GCP.

The international harmonisation process (ICH) led by the three major world pharmaceutical markets, the USA, Europe and Japan, began in 1990 and continues even now. New, international GCP Guidelines, as already mentioned, came into effect in January 1997 and define the one common standard to which clinical researchers world-wide should adhere.

The consequences of GCP are that the data obtained are of a higher quality and the patients and volunteers participating in clinical trials are better protected. However, GCP has undoubtedly introduced a greater administrative burden and consequently higher costs and more staff are involved.

GOOD CLINICAL PRACTICE – WHAT IS IT?

The basic principles of GCP are firstly: protection of the patient or volunteer and secondly: that the data obtained are correct and reproducible.

In addition to the European Community Guidelines, the Scandinavian countries, the World Health Organisation, the US Food and Drug Administration and the Association of the British Pharmaceutical Industry all introduced guidelines and regulations for performing clinical trials. Often there are also national laws to adhere to.

In Europe the guidelines for GCP were contained in the document 'Good Clinical Practice for Trials on Medicinal Products in the European Community'. Not all of the document applies directly to Investigators, but certain sections are pivotal to your work as an Investigator in clinical trials. From January 1997, the European Guidelines have been superseded by the ICH GCP Guidelines and these must be your terms of reference for all clinical trials conducted at your study site.

Here follows a summary of the European GCP Guidelines, with emphasis on the parts which are relevant to your function as Investigator. These are reproduced here to emphasise that GCP is not new. The defined obligations in the conduct of trials go back to 1991 or earlier when European GCP was introduced.

The document is divided into five chapters, with a Glossary and an Appendix.

The list of Abbreviations is a useful quick reference for terms which you will often encounter in the field of clinical trials.

Chapter 1 deals with the protection of trial subjects and consultation of Ethics Committees. All people engaged in clinical research must know and follow the ethical guidelines in the most up-to-date revision of the Declaration of Helsinki. Also 'The personal integrity and welfare of the trial subjects is the ultimate responsibility of the Investigator in relation to the trial'. There are then listed details regarding Ethics Committees and informed consent. These will be dealt with in the respective SOP.

Chapter 2 deals with the responsibilities of three of the main parties in clinical studies: the Sponsor, the Monitor and the Investigator.

* The Sponsor's responsibilities include the selection of Investigators, informing the Investigators, notification of the relevant authorities, provision and documentation of study medication, adverse event reporting, compensation for injury or death for the subjects on a trial, and indemnity for the Investigator.
* The Monitor's main responsibility is to be the main communication link between the Sponsor and the Investigator. The other responsibilities include working according to SOPs and visiting the Investigator before, during and after the trial to check that the trial is being conducted correctly. This includes comparing the case report form (CRF) entries with source documents.
* The responsibilities of the Investigator will be summarised below, but they are included in each SOP as appropriate – *if you work according to properly prepared SOPs as well as the highest medical standards you will be conducting your clinical trials in accordance with GCP.* In contrast to the Sponsor and Monitor, it is not a responsibility of the Investigator to work according to SOPs. However it will certainly simplify your work if you do.

RESPONSIBILITIES OF THE INVESTIGATOR

* The Investigator must be familiar with the properties of the study medication – this information will be found in the Investigator's Brochure provided by the Sponsor.
* You must have sufficient time and resources to conduct the trial, including patient resources.
* An up-to-date curriculum vitae must be submitted to the Sponsor.
* The protocol must be signed, confirming that you have read it, understood it and will work according to it.
* If appropriate, you can nominate a local study Co-ordinator to assist with the administration of the trial. This will depend on the requirements of the trial and obviously the resources of the study centre.
* Other involved staff members must be informed about the trial, as must local hospital management and the institute/local/regional Ethics Committee.
* Informed consent must be obtained from each patient/volunteer.

- Drug accountability is a term which you will encounter when you perform a trial according to GCP Guidelines. Drug accountability means knowing and keeping records of the exact whereabouts of study medication, including delivery, storage, dispensing and returns from patients.
- In double blind trials there is always an accompanying coding procedure, so that in an emergency you can find out which drug the patient has been receiving. This may only be done in accordance with the procedure in the protocol and must be documented. The Monitor must also be consulted or informed when this is done.
- All data relating to the clinical trial must be collected, recorded and reported properly.
- An important area of clinical trials is the assessment and procedures relating to adverse events. Full details will be provided in the SOP section.
- Any data relevant to the study must be made available to the Sponsor of the trial, the Monitor and any other relevant authority for verification, audit or inspection.
- All case report forms, analyses and reports must be signed by you, including the final report of the trial.
- You should also remember that all information obtained in the course of the trial is to be kept strictly confidential. This applies not only to information relating to patients and volunteers, but also to information supplied by the Sponsor, some of which may be commercially sensitive.
- There are several points relating to patient care for patients taking part in clinical trials – these are listed in SOP 1: Study Organisation and Planning.

Chapter 3 deals with data handling by the Sponsor including archiving of data, **Chapter 4** with statistics and **Chapter 5** with Quality Assurance.

The Appendix provides guidance on some of the practical aspects of clinical trials and includes a useful section on the content of a trial protocol and case report forms.

The ICH GCP Guidelines follow a different format. After the introduction there are eight sections which include a useful glossary. **Section 4** is the principal section relating to the Investigator, although unlike the European GCP Guidelines there are aspects of several sections which impact on the Investigator and his or her team. A most important difference from the European GCP Guidelines is covered in **Section 8** in which the essential documents for the conduct of a clinical trial are noted. This contains full details of those documents that must be retained in the Investigator's Study File at the study site. The ICH GCP Guidelines are generally considered more comprehensive than the European predecessor, and need no additional summary here.

STANDARD OPERATING PROCEDURES

What are Standard Operating Procedures?

SOPs are defined in the ICH GCP Guidelines as 'detailed, written instructions to achieve uniformity of the performance of a specific function'.

As mentioned above, it is not a GCP requirement that you, as an Investigator, work according to SOPs (unless you are also acting as the Sponsor for the trial). However, as you can see from the list of Investigator responsibilities above, there are many facets to performing a clinical trial apart from the clinical/medical aspects. The aim of these SOPs and accompanying checklists is to simplify the organisation and documentation of clinical trials, whilst maintaining high standards of Good Clinical Practice.

SOPs should be detailed enough so that a procedure can be correctly carried out in a reproducible manner, but not so specific that they can only be applied to one clinical trial and then have to be rewritten for the next. It is almost always necessary to adapt SOPs to an individual hospital or department, and the SOPs here can be tailored to suit your needs, as long as the requirements of GCP are maintained.

The SOPs here can be broadly divided into the following sections:

General study organisation
Pre-study
During study
End of study

The general outline of an SOP is as follows:

Number and title of procedure
Purpose (brief summary in a few lines)
Other procedures simultaneously involved
Personnel involved and procedure: **Who** is responsible for carrying out the procedure?
When and **How** should the procedure be carried out?
Date of version in use plus 'replaces previous version of . . .'
Name of author and person in charge who approved this version

Each SOP has a number. Not every SOP has an accompanying checklist. Please note that the checklists are numbered according to the corresponding SOP number.

Revision and updating of Standard Operating Procedures

SOPs must be reviewed and updated on a regular basis. When they are first introduced to the department, they may need revision after a few months. However, once they have been adjusted to your needs they will probably only need revising every two years or so, but we recommend an annual review.

Revision is best done as a team task. The procedures should be examined and rewritten where appropriate, then approved and signed. The old version should be archived. It should not be disposed of because it can be some time after a study is completed that Regulatory Agency questions might arise, and you may be required to show the procedures you used to follow.

ORGANISATION OF CLINICAL TRIALS

Pharmaceutical company as Sponsor

Because of financial pressures, clinical research involving new products has generally moved away from independent research based in teaching hospitals and university departments, towards research where a pharmaceutical company acts as a Sponsor. In addition, it is often not practical that doctors working in a busy hospital take on not only their responsibilities as Investigators, but also the responsibilities of the Sponsor with the related administration and organisation.

The increased costs in clinical research are largely related to the introduction of GCP standards – for purely financial reasons fully implemented GCP is often considered practical only when a trial is sponsored by the pharmaceutical industry. Therefore the SOPs and checklists written here are based on such arrangements. If you are acting as Sponsor/Investigator, please read the section below.

Investigator as Sponsor

If you are planning on performing a study with no external Sponsor, you have many responsibilities in addition to those which you have as an Investigator. As stated above, the SOPs written here are intended for Investigators who are working together with a Sponsor.

Basically the additional responsibilities include notification of and/or obtaining approval from the relevant authorities before the study start, provision and documentation of study medication, adverse event reporting, and providing compensation for injury or death for the subjects on a trial.

If you are performing your study according to GCP (and in many countries this already is, or will become, a legal requirement) you must be prepared to invest much time and effort in the study.

Working with Contract Research Organisations

Contract Research Organisations (CROs) are institutions employing anything from one to several thousand people and are involved in performing clinical research on a contract basis for a pharmaceutical company. This means they are contracted by pharmaceutical companies to perform some or all of their duties as Sponsor for a clinical trial. For example a CRO may be contracted to perform just the monitoring of the trial, or the statistical analysis, or write the protocol, etc. CROs are often contracted to cover the periods when the pharmaceutical company has no spare personnel. However, it can also be that the CRO has specialised local knowledge, particularly in international, multi-centre trials.

If a CRO is working on a trial together with a Sponsor, make sure you know exactly which person you should contact when. It may be that for randomisation you should contact the CRO, but for the reporting of serious adverse events you should contact the Sponsor.

REFERENCES

1. ICH SECRETARIAT (1996). *ICH Harmonised Tripartite Guideline for Good Clinical Practice.* IFPMA, Geneva.
2. POCOCK, S. J. (1983). *Clinical Trials: A Practical Approach.* John Wiley & Sons.
3. LOCK, S. & WELLS, F. (Eds) (1993). *Fraud and Misconduct in Medical Research.* BMJ Publishing Group.
4. CPMP WORKING PARTY (1991). *Good Clinical Practice for Trials on Medicinal Products in the European Community.* CPMP Working Party on Efficacy of Medicinal Products, Commission of European Communities, Brussels. Document 111/3976/88-EN (Final).
5. HUTT, P. B. (1993). The Regulation of Pharmaceutical Products in the USA. In: D. M. BURLEY, J. M. CLARKE & L. LASAGNA (Eds), *Pharmaceutical Medicine.* Edward Arnold.

Abbreviations

AE
Adverse Event

AMG
Arzneimittelgesetz (German term for Medicines Law)

CRA
Clinical Research Associate or Clinical Research Assistant
Another term for Monitor

CRF
Case Report Form or Case Record Form

FDA
Food and Drug Administration

GCP
Good Clinical Practice

GLP
Good Laboratory Practice

GMP
Good Manufacturing Practice

ICH
International Conference on Harmonisation

IND
Investigational New Drug

IRB
Institutional Review Board, the FDA term for an Ethics Committee

SAE
Serious Adverse Event

SDV
Source Data Verification or Source Document Verification

SOP
Standard Operating Procedure

SOP 0
Preparation, Approval and Review of SOPs

Background

The ICH GCP Guidelines consolidate the European Guidelines on Good Clinical Practice, in which the first responsibility of the Sponsor was to 'establish detailed Standard Operating Procedures (SOPs) to comply with Good Clinical Practice'. There is no such similar requirement for the Investigator, even in the ICH GCP Guidelines. However, the use of Standard Operating Procedures within clinical and laboratory research undoubtedly leads to increased uniformity of method and consequent reproducibility of results. Clinical study sites in possession of well documented good Standard Operating Procedures detailing the way in which work is or will be conducted at the study site will find that potential Sponsors consider this to be a good feature of the site. SOPs assist in the training and management of new and temporary staff and help ensure between-trial uniformity where a series of studies is conducted.

SOPs, when they are in place, will be documents against which the site's performance will be judged in the event of an audit. Failure to follow SOPs is a reason for failing an audit. SOPs, therefore, should reflect the true practice at the site and not be a set of idealistic rules or guidelines that can be followed only when particular conditions prevail. For this reason, it is commonly recognised that the best person to write an SOP is the person who carries out the procedure. This is not essential, however, but a useful tip. What is essential is that the individuals having to carry out the procedure are satisfied that it works in practice all the time or almost all the time.

There will always be new and unforeseen problems and from time to time the occurrence of one will highlight a weakness in an SOP. This should not be seen as a major problem, merely an indication of the need for a revision to an SOP. SOPs identified as inadequate should generally be revised as soon as possible, but if the change is not immediate, then the details of the problem should be recorded so that the appropriate changes can be made at the next review. Records of SOP deviations and actions taken should be kept to assist any auditor in future.

SOPs can become outdated without staff even becoming aware, if a procedure tends to be followed without reference to the printed SOPs and the procedure changes subtly. A periodic review of SOPs is highly recommended; an annual review is usually considered acceptable in the pharmaceutical industry and we recommend the same for site SOPs. However, it may be wise when first implementing SOPs for them to be reviewed sooner than this the first time. Old versions of SOPs should be maintained with dates of effectiveness so that work is audited against the appropriate document, not merely the most recent, which could well lead to unnecessary failure.

SOP 0
Preparation, Approval and Review of SOPs

SOPs should be formally approved and generally this should be by an individual other than the author. The nature of clinical trials is such that ultimate responsibility at the study site lies with the Principal Investigator and consequently he or she should approve all SOPs. Depending on the size and scope of the study site it may be sensible to have more than one authorising signatory and a valid SOP in this case should be signed off by all such individuals. For the purpose of the SOP that follows, however, a single authorising signatory, namely the Investigator, is assumed.

SOP 0
Preparation, Approval and Review of SOPs

Purpose

To describe the procedure for preparing, approving and distributing SOPs in the department. To describe the procedure for dealing with identified revisions and for conduct of regular review of SOPs.

Other Related Procedures

All SOPs

Procedure

1. Who?

The Investigator or other named individual, if this task is delegated, is responsible for ensuring that Standard Operating Procedures are prepared, reviewed, revised and approved according to the required procedure. The same people are responsible for ensuring that the author of each SOP is adequately placed to prepare a reasonable document.

The Investigator is responsible for authorising the content of each SOP.

2. When?

Before the conduct of each trial the SOPs to which the trial will be conducted should be up to date.

Deficiencies requiring SOP amendments should be dealt with at the earliest opportunity but no later than the next SOP review.

SOPs should be reviewed three months after the first implementation and annually thereafter.

3. How?

- All SOPs should be prepared according to a standard format, which should be defined (an example is the style used here and in other SOPs in this book).
- Each SOP should be prepared (authored) by someone competent to do so and eventually signed off by that individual.
- Each SOP should be reviewed at draft stage by staff who will use it and identified deficiencies addressed.

SOP 0
Preparation, Approval and Review of SOPs

- Each SOP should be reviewed by the Investigator, and once satisfied that it is adequate, the Investigator should authorise it by signing it off.
- Each SOP should show the date of preparation (i.e. when signed off by the author), the date of approval (i.e. when signed off by the Investigator) and the date it is effective from.
- Each SOP should indicate whether it replaces a previous version and, if so, which.
- All new SOPs should be reviewed for accuracy three–six months after first implementation.
- All existing SOPs will be reviewed annually at a time specified.
- Deficiencies identified in SOPs will be recorded and appropriate SOPs prepared or existing ones modified to address the deficiencies.

SOP approved by: _____

Signature: _____ *Date:* _____

SOP 0 – CHECKLIST
Preparation, Approval and Review of SOPs

This form should be initiated when need for a new SOP is identified. It should be passed to the individual who will prepare the SOP and circulated with draft versions of the new SOP for review and comment. Comments should be written on the draft document or elsewhere and returned to the originator with the form duly completed. The form should remain with the SOP until the first review is completed.

Title of proposed new SOP _____

To be prepared by whom? _____

Draft to be circulated by when? _____ *dd/mm/yy*

Draft to go to whom? _____

_____

To be returned to _____ *by when* _____ *dd/mm/yy*

                                              Comments?

Reviewed by   _____

                       dd/mm/yy   *y/n*

                       _____

                       dd/mm/yy   *y/n*

                       _____

                       dd/mm/yy   *y/n*

Summary of action taken following comments

_____

_____

Further draft required?   *Y/N*   *If yes, circulate with revised version of form.*

*Date SOP finalised*_____ *dd/mm/yy*

*Date SOP approved*_____ *dd/mm/yy*

*Date of first scheduled review*_____ *dd/mm/yy*

*When carried out?*_____ *dd/mm/yy*

By whom? _____

SOP revised?   *Y/N*

SOP 0 – CHECKLIST
Preparation, Approval and Review of SOPs

This form should be used for the annual review of SOPs. Scheduled date of review mm/yy

SOPs	Reviewer initials	Changes Y/N	Date Revised dd/mm/yy
SOP 0. Preparation, approval and review of SOPs			
SOP 1. Study organisation and planning			
SOP 2. Study team – definition of responsibilities			
SOP 3. Study files and filing			
SOP 4. Local management requirements			
SOP 5. Review and validation of the protocol			
SOP 6. Review of protocol amendments			
SOP 7. Case Report Form (CRF) review			
SOP 8. Investigator's Brochure			
SOP 9. Estimation of patient numbers			
SOP 10. Ethics Committee			
SOP 11. Indemnity, compensation and insurance			
SOP 12. Laboratory			
SOP 13. Pre-study monitoring visits			
SOP 14. Patient recruitment and intention to enrol			
SOP 15. Obtaining personal written informed consent			
SOP 16. Obtaining informed consent for patients unable to give personal consent			
SOP 17. Randomisation and stratification			
SOP 18. Blinding: codes and code breaking			
SOP 19. Case Report Form (CRF) completion			
SOP 20. Study drugs			
SOP 21. Monitoring visits			
SOP 22. Adverse events and serious adverse event reporting			
SOP 23. Nursing procedures			
SOP 24. Clinical procedures			
SOP 25. Trial report			
SOP 26. Archiving			
SOP 27. Audits and inspections			

SOP 0 – CHECKLIST
Preparation, Approval and Review of SOPs

This form should be completed whenever a deficiency in an SOP is identified and maintained with the SOP until an authorised replacement is in place.

SOP number _____ Version number _____

Details of problem or deficiency in SOP _____

_____

_____

_____

Identified by _____ Date: dd/mm/yy

Discussed with _____

SOP revision required   y/n   If yes, to be carried out by whom? _____

If no, why not? _____

Date SOP re-finalised   dd/mm/yy

Date SOP approved   dd/mm/yy

SOP 1
Study Organisation and Planning

Background

This procedure should be applied to every study conducted in the department. It should be used by all members of the department working on the study to co-ordinate procedures. It will aid the selection of other SOPs for use with specific aspects of the study.

A study organisation checklist will act as a guide to the SOPs and checklists necessary for the particular study. Several SOPs and checklists must be referred to for every study – for example, every study will need Ethics Committee review. However, if the study is not blinded, clearly you don't need to refer to the Blinding SOP. A specimen study flowchart is shown on the following page.

The flowchart is intended to help as a reminder of the various considerations that might apply in each clinical trial and to put them in perspective with each other. The diagram is not a true flowchart in that several procedures may be performed simultaneously, if appropriate. The flowchart can be adapted to take account of specific local or therapeutic area requirements.

SOP 1
Study Organisation and Planning

Study Flowchart

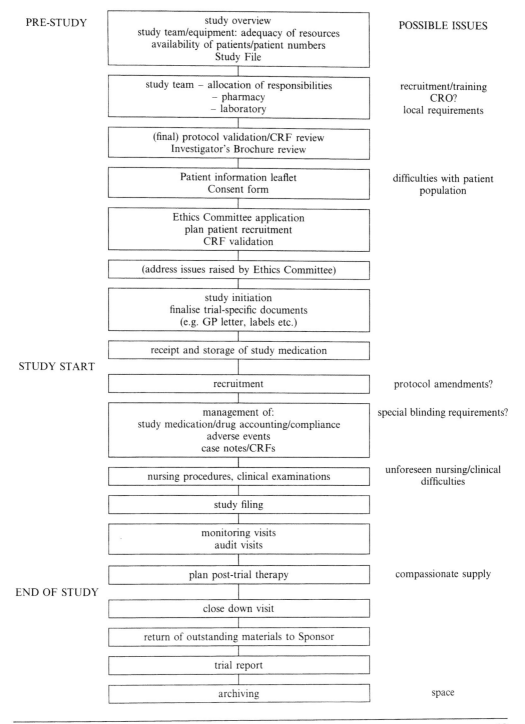

PRE-STUDY

POSSIBLE ISSUES

| study overview |
| study team/equipment: adequacy of resources |
| availability of patients/patient numbers |
| Study File |

| study team – allocation of responsibilities |
| – pharmacy |
| – laboratory |

recruitment/training
CRO?
local requirements

| (final) protocol validation/CRF review |
| Investigator's Brochure review |

| Patient information leaflet |
| Consent form |

difficulties with patient
population

| Ethics Committee application |
| plan patient recruitment |
| CRF validation |

| (address issues raised by Ethics Committee) |

| study initiation |
| finalise trial-specific documents |
| (e.g. GP letter, labels etc.) |

| receipt and storage of study medication |

STUDY START

| recruitment |

protocol amendments?

| management of: |
| study medication/drug accounting/compliance |
| adverse events |
| case notes/CRFs |

special blinding requirements?

| nursing procedures, clinical examinations |

unforeseen nursing/clinical
difficulties

| study filing |

| monitoring visits |
| audit visits |

| plan post-trial therapy |

compassionate supply

END OF STUDY

| close down visit |

| return of outstanding materials to Sponsor |

| trial report |

| archiving |

space

SOP 1
Study Organisation and Planning

Purpose

To provide an overview for the organisation and planning of each clinical trial performed in the department. To identify key activities and responsibilities.

Other Related Procedures

All SOPs

Procedure

1. Who?

It remains the final responsibility of the Principal Investigator to ensure that the study is performed according to GCP and national guidelines and legal requirements. This responsibility cannot be transferred.

Each study will be the day to day responsibility of one nominated member of the department. The nominated individual will be documented in the Study File. For sponsored trials, the Sponsor will be informed of the name and contact details of the individual responsible for the study and will usually be asked to address or copy all written information to that person. If this individual is not the Investigator, the responsibility for the study will be jointly that of the individual and the Investigator and ultimate responsibility for the trial rests with the Investigator.

For sponsored trials, the individuals at the site involved with the study and their roles and responsibilities should be documented and made known to the Sponsor. Details of relevant individuals acting on behalf of the Sponsor should be noted in the Study File.

2. When?

This SOP is the reference for all other SOPs and should be referred to when required at any stage in the study.

The individual responsible for the study should be nominated as early as possible and preferably no later than when it seems likely the study will proceed to Ethics Committee application.

For all trials, names and roles of individuals involved in the study should be agreed no later than the start of the study, defined, for the purposes of this SOP as the granting of Ethics Committee approval or a later date agreed with the Sponsor, where there is one.

For all trials, after the initial introduction of the study (the first pre-study meeting or the first draft protocol), a study organisation checklist should be completed.

SOP 1
Study Organisation and Planning

3. How?

Pre-study procedures

- Complete a study organisation checklist.
- Allocate responsibilities to the study team.
- Set up a Study File. Request assistance from the Sponsor if necessary.
- Ensure arrangements for pre-study meetings are made.
- Ensure adequate review of the study protocol, and/or CRFs/diary cards and Investigator's Brochure as available.
- File key documents: CVs, laboratory reference ranges and provide copies to the Sponsor when one exists. File in the Study File all relevant documents forwarded by the Sponsor.
- Ethical aspects of the study must be taken care of:
  - review and agree informed consent procedure and material
  - inform Sponsor of Ethics Committee requirements
  - prepare Ethics Committee submission
  - obtain Ethics Committee review.
- Overall numbers of patients and the number at this centre must be agreed.
- The procedure for patient recruitment must be reviewed and the likely number of patients recruited in what time period estimated.
- The procedure for randomisation and stratification must be established.
- Review terms and conditions: indemnity, arrangements for compensating subjects in the event of injury, financial agreements, publication, registration with the authorities, division of responsibilities with a Sponsor.
- Carry out any specific requirements of the local management (e.g. hospital management or health authority). Specific requirements applying to all trials at this centre should be detailed in an SOP drawn up for the purpose.
- Assess laboratory (including external labs) and Pharmacy requirements.
- Assess staffing, equipment and space requirements.
- Make arrangements for receipt and storage of study medication.
- Before enrolment of the first patient ensure all involved staff are familiar with the protocol (and if applicable the Investigator's Brochure), with completing the CRFs, and with the procedure for reporting adverse events.
- Ensure also that the appropriate staff are familiar with the arrangements for drug accountability, and any special, study-specific, clinical or nursing procedures.
- A study initiation meeting should take place and its details recorded and filed.
- Thought should be given at the beginning of the trial to the archiving requirements that might be necessary and to any special post-trial therapy requirements of the patients.

SOP 1
Study Organisation and Planning

Procedures to be carried out during the trial

During the trial, the pre-trial procedures (above) should be referred to as and when necessary. In particular, if the protocol is amended, the pre-trial requirements of this SOP should be reviewed to determine follow-up actions.

- Hold study meetings within the department as required to discuss study progress and maintain interest in the study.
- For sponsored trials, provide information on the progress of the study as reasonably requested by the Sponsor. Inform the Sponsor of difficulties that may impinge on the progress of the study at the earliest opportunity.
- For sponsored trials, assist the Sponsor's representatives with monitoring, audit and other visits.
- Provide progress reports according to local requirements (e.g. Ethics Committee, local management). These requirements should be detailed in a specific SOP.
- Liaise with other departments involved with the trial to ensure that any concerns are dealt with efficiently (e.g. Pharmacy, laboratories).
- Prior to the end of the trial agree archiving arrangements (with Sponsor if applicable).
- Prior to the completion of the first patient in the trial consider any special requirements for post-trial therapy.

End of trial

- Ensure study is formally closed down and appropriate bodies notified.
- Archive study documents as agreed (with Sponsor if applicable).
- Ensure return of any study material required by the Sponsor.
- The trial report (provided it is made available, probably some months later) should be reviewed and approved, in writing. If it cannot be approved, this is acceptable, but should be documented.

General points

Other general points from the EC Guidelines affecting study organisation and documentation include:

- Depending on the nature of the trial, fully functional resuscitation equipment should be immediately available in case of emergency.
- The Principal Investigator (or possibly a Co-Investigator) is medically responsible for the patient/volunteer under his or her care for the duration of the trial and must also ensure that appropriate medical care is available after the trial. Even when there has been a good response to the study medication, the study medication may not be available to the patient at the end of the clinical trial.

Study Organisation and Planning

- Clinically significant abnormal laboratory values or clinical observations must be followed up after the trial.
- If the trial involves out-patients, they should be provided with an identification card stating that they are taking part in a clinical trial, with relevant contact addresses and telephone numbers. Medical records should also clearly indicate the subject's participation in the trial and the family doctor should be informed, with the agreement of the subject.

SOP approved by: _____

Signature: _____ *Date:* _____

SOP 1 – CHECKLIST
Study Organisation and Planning

Protocol Code: [   ]   Date of Protocol: | | | |
                                                    dd mm yy

Abbreviated Title: _____

Sponsor Name: _____

This checklist should be completed when the first version of the protocol has been reviewed or after the initial pre-trial meeting, whichever is sooner. Complete every field (N/A if not applicable – do not leave blank). Complete further copies of the checklist as required.

Protocol available (from Sponsor)? (✓) Yes ( ) No ( ). Date if Yes: _____

Pre-trial meeting held (with Sponsor)? (✓) Yes ( ) No ( ). Date if Yes: _____

Protocol Details

(Sponsor's) Protocol Reference Number: _____

Full Title:

Date of Protocol: _____

Date signed by Principal Investigator: _____

Study Details

Dates: Planned Ethics Committee Meeting:
                              Planned Start:
                           End Recruitment:
        End of Treatment Period – Last Patient:
                              End of Study:

Investigator/Centre ID:
(allocated by Sponsor)

SOP 1 – CHECKLIST
Study Organisation and Planning

Name and address of Sponsor: (If self-sponsored, then fill in Investigator's details)

Name _____

Name of contact   Dr/Mr/Ms _____   _____
                            Forename   Surname

Position   _____

Address   _____
           _____
           _____
           _____

Telephone   _____

Fax   _____

Monitor Details (if different):   **Not Applicable? ( )**

Name   Dr/Mr/Ms _____   _____
                 Forename   Surname

Address   _____
           _____
           _____
           _____

Telephone   _____

Fax   _____

Contract Research Organisation Details: Not Applicable? ( )

Name   _____

Name of contact   Dr/Mr/Ms _____   _____
                            Forename   Surname

Address   _____
           _____
           _____
           _____

Telephone   _____

Fax   _____

Checklist completed by: _____ *on* _____
                                                            (date)

SOP 2
Study Team: Definition of Responsibilities

Background

Definitions from the EC Guidelines:

An Investigator is one or more persons responsible for the practical performance of a trial and for the integrity, health and welfare of the subjects during the trial.

He/she must be:

- Appropriately qualified and legally allowed to practise medicine or dentistry
- Trained and experienced in research, particularly in the clinical area of the proposed trial
- Familiar with the background to and the requirements of the study
- Known to have high ethical standards and professional integrity.

There are, however, no precise definitions of the required qualifications. For a Principal Investigator, the following can be used as an additional guide:

- At least two years' experience of working as an Investigator in clinical studies for the particular indication
- Experience in procedures for adverse event detection, reporting and treatment
- Trained in GCP (with certification, where possible).

Please note the difference between the definition used in the EC Guidelines for the Principal Investigator and the definition used in these SOPs. In the EC Guidelines the Principal Investigator is defined as the Investigator responsible for the co-ordination of the Investigators at the different centres. In these SOPs the Principal Investigator is defined as the Investigator taking overall responsibility for the study at the department. All other Investigators in the same department are Co-Investigators or Sub-Investigators according to ICH GCP. The term 'Investigators' refers to the Principal Investigator and all Co-Investigators.

The EC Guidelines define the term Study Co-ordinator (local) as 'an appropriately experienced person nominated by the Investigator to assist administering the trial at the investigational site'. In these SOPs the Co-ordinator will be referred to as the Study Site Co-ordinator, abbreviated to SSC. In smaller trials, or in departments where such staff do not exist, or in other areas where appropriate, these tasks may be allocated to one of the Co-Investigators or taken on by the Principal Investigator.

SOP 2
Study Team: Definition of Responsibilities

Purpose

To assist in the division and allocation of responsibilities within the study team at the department, to ensure smooth running of the trial. To provide the Sponsor with an overview of the division of responsibilities within the trial.

Other Related Procedures

All SOPs

Procedure

1. Who?

During the pre-study phase, the Principal Investigator and the individual responsible for the trial must discuss and agree on the study requirements with the Monitor of the trial. The types of tasks that can be delegated will depend on the suitability of the individuals to accept the tasks.

2. When?

The initial allocation of responsibilities is one of the first tasks in the pre-study phase.

3. How?

- Each trial will have a Principal Investigator, who has overall responsibility for:
  - the welfare of the patients
  - conduct of the study in the department
  - administration of drugs
  - ensuring that local management needs are met
  - ensuring that Ethics Committee requirements are met.
- The Principal Investigator should, where required, allocate day to day responsibility to one member of the department.
- The study responsible person should, with the Principal Investigator where required, discuss and agree the allocation of tasks with the staff members. The allocation of tasks should be recorded (for example, on the checklist attached).
- Where one exists, an external Sponsor should be made aware of the planned division of tasks. Contact names and roles of other individuals involved with the trial (e.g. Pharmacy, laboratory staff) should also be notified to the Sponsor.

SOP 2
Study Team: Definition of Responsibilities

- The study responsible person, with the Principal Investigator where required, should appraise the need for additional staff, and discuss changes with the Sponsor where there is one.
- Where there is a medically qualified Co-Investigator, he or she may normally:
  - take informed consent
  - sign prescriptions
  - sign off Case Record Forms
  - conduct clinical examinations, evaluate laboratory and other reports and carry out any other assessments of a medical nature.

Unless otherwise specified in writing, a Study Site Co-ordinator or Study Nurse will not normally conduct these activities, though assistance with them may be given.

SOP approved by: _____

Signature: _____ *Date:* _____

SOP 2 – CHECKLIST
Study Team: Definition of Responsibilities

Protocol Code: [_____]   Date of Protocol: |__|__|__|
                                                dd mm yy

Abbreviated Title: _____

Sponsor Name: _____

Who of the following will be in the study team?

	Number	Name	Enter each individual only once in the most appropriate role

Principal Investigator   [1]

Co-Investigator(s)   [ ]

Study Site Co-ordinator(s)   [ ]

Study Nurse(s)   [ ]

Laboratory   [ ]

Pharmacy   [ ]

Other _____   [ ]

Team Member	Name	Specimen Signature	Initials	Tel/Pager Numbers
Principal Investigator			|__|__|	
Other: _____			|__|__|	
_____			|__|__|	

Continue on a second sheet if required

SOP 2 – CHECKLIST
Study Team: Definition of Responsibilities

Study Organisation and Allocation of Responsibilities

	Yes	No	Details
Have general arrangements been made for holiday cover and night and weekend duties? If yes, give details. If no, give reasons or intentions.	☐	☐	_____ _____

Pre-ticked items apply to all trials. Add extra ticks for items applicable to this trial, e.g. 'randomisation'.

Check through the table and tick all procedures necessary for the study. Allocate responsibilities and enter individuals' initials in the table.

Activity	When	required?	initials lead person	others
Study organisation/study team*	pre-	✓	⊔⊔	⊔⊔
Study File set up and management	pre-	✓	⊔⊔	⊔⊔
Financial agreement	pre-		⊔⊔	⊔⊔
Indemnity, compensation and insurance	pre-	✓	⊔⊔	⊔⊔
Protocol approval*	pre-	✓	⊔⊔	⊔⊔
CRF approval*	pre-		⊔⊔	⊔⊔
Investigator's Brochure/product information	pre-		⊔⊔	⊔⊔
Patient numbers*	pre-	✓	⊔⊔	⊔⊔
Ethics Committee*	pre-	✓	⊔⊔	⊔⊔
Laboratory*	pre-		⊔⊔	⊔⊔
Pharmacy*	pre-		⊔⊔	⊔⊔
Pre-study visits*	pre-	✓	⊔⊔	⊔⊔
Patient recruitment strategy*	pre-	✓	⊔⊔	⊔⊔
Patient information and consent*	pre-	✓	⊔⊔	⊔⊔
Randomisation	during		⊔⊔	⊔⊔
Blinding	during		⊔⊔	⊔⊔
CRF completion	during	✓	⊔⊔	⊔⊔
Study medication – receipt and storage	pre-	✓	⊔⊔	⊔⊔
Drug accountability and monitoring of compliance	during	✓	⊔⊔	⊔⊔
Monitoring visits*	during	✓	⊔⊔	⊔⊔

SOP 2 – CHECKLIST
Study Team: Definition of Responsibilities

Adverse events	during	✓	⊔⊔	⊔⊔
Nursing procedures	during		⊔⊔	⊔⊔
Clinical examinations	during		⊔⊔	⊔⊔
Audits and inspections	during		⊔⊔	⊔⊔
Return of study supplies	end	✓	⊔⊔	⊔⊔
Trial report*	end	✓	⊔⊔	⊔⊔
Post-study therapy	before end		⊔⊔	⊔⊔
Archiving*	before end	✓	⊔⊔	⊔⊔

* denotes that a checklist should also be completed.

Checklist completed by: _____ *on* _____
                                                              (date)

SOP 3
Study Files and Filing

Background

With the large volume of documentation required for each trial a satisfactory filing system is necessary. Where there is an external Sponsor, it is likely the department will be provided with a Study File for each individual trial, but by the time it arrives there may well be a considerable quantity of documentation already associated with the trial. A standard procedure for each trial taking account of an external Sponsor's likely filing arrangement should mean fewer mistakes will be made and documents will be easier to find, both whilst the trial is in progress and once the documentation has been archived.

Pharmaceutical Sponsors and CROs providing Study Files generally have a standard file with sub-divisions that are similar from Sponsor to Sponsor. Sub-division of the site file in advance along the same lines will make re-filing into the Sponsor's file easier.

One point to note is that financial agreements could previously be filed separately, away from the Study File, but as a requirement of ICH GCP they must now be in the Study File.

SOP 3
Study Files and Filing

Purpose

To describe the procedure for the filing of study documentation.

Other Related Procedures

SOP 26: Archiving

Procedure

1. Who?

The person who has been delegated the responsibility for the general organisation of the study, together with the person assigned to setting up and monitoring the Study File, must ensure that the necessary files are established and properly maintained.

2. When?

A Study File should be prepared as soon as is practical after the first contact by the Sponsor, or for trials where there is no separate Sponsor, as soon as an outline protocol is available. The file should be actively maintained from this time until the trial is formally closed (by the Sponsor if applicable). When it becomes available, the final report should be lodged with the Study File.

3. How?

- Specific space will be allotted for the filing of prospective studies, where protocols and Investigator's Brochures and early correspondence can be stored when they are first produced or received by the department.
- The filing system should be segmented so that individual trials remain separate. Further segmentation within each trial will be essential at a later date, but is not necessary initially.
- If the Principal Investigator decides that the department will not participate in the study, the protocol and Investigator's Brochure should be returned in the case of an external Sponsor.

If the study is to proceed, a 'Study File' will be established. The protocol and Investigator's Brochure and all other accumulated material should be transferred to this study-specific file. The file will be labelled with the protocol number but not the title of the study. The telephone number of the Sponsor and a contact name should also appear on the label, or on the cover of the folder. This enables the Sponsor to be contacted swiftly if required by individuals less familiar with the trial.

SOP 3
Study Files and Filing

The Study File will be sub-divided. For example:

- Correspondence.
- Protocol and Amendments.
- Investigator's Brochure.
- Drug accountability.
- Ethics Committee.
- List of patients entered (to enable easy identification of individuals in the future. The list should also include those actively considered for the trial but not entered, with reasons for non-entry where appropriate).
- Code envelopes may be stored in the Study File, but may be stored separately, e.g. at Pharmacy. The location should be recorded.
- Where required, registration of clinical trial with the regulatory authorities and/or local management.
- Completed serious adverse event forms (if not included in the CRFs).
- Financial agreement, unless stored elsewhere.
- Records of telephone conversations and notes of study meetings should also be filed. The Sponsor will also keep records of telephone conversations and make written reports after each visit. During an audit, these records will be checked for consistency.
- Completed consent forms (or copies).
- Study-specific SOP checklists.
- The completed CRFs will usually be stored in a separate file.

A Study File may consist of more than one distinct file. Too many different files should be avoided. It is usually unnecessary that each individual patient has a separate file. The Investigator's Brochure may also need to be located separately; if so, the Study File should indicate where.

Each patient's informed consent form should be filed in the patient's medical notes.

Filing source documents

Study data which is to be supported by source documents must be defined.

Source documents must be traceable. If documents are routinely stored separately from the patient's notes, e.g. radiographs, and they belong to the source data, then a note should be made in the Study File or in the other source documents as to where the other documents are stored. If there are several such documents, it may be necessary to complete a table for each, documenting where they can be found (see Figure 1).

SOP 3
Study Files and Filing

Figure 1. Example for Tracing Source Documents

Patient number: _____ Study number: _____

Document	Date of assessment	Location where stored	Contact person/ telephone number
ECG			
Histology report			
Radiograph			

SOP approved by: _____

Signature: _____ *Date:* _____

SOP 4
Local Management Requirements

Background

In addition to the GCP Guidelines and any national laws relating to clinical studies, there may also exist guidelines specific to the particular study site, be this hospital, general practice surgery or other 'site'. These may be, for example, requirements of the local health authority, or equivalent, or of the management of the institution. Such requirements may relate to Ethics Committee approval, registration of the trial with management or a Research Committee, signing of clinical trial indemnity or approval of financial agreements.

The generation of a template SOP for requirements that are site-specific is impossible in this manual. We encourage each centre to generate one or more specific SOPs to cover the standard local requirements that apply to all, or the majority of, trials. We suggest using the layout used in the SOPs presented elsewhere in this manual, but if a more convenient way exists for a specific local requirement, there is nothing to stop a different format being followed.

SOPs worth considering are, for example:

- Application for Ethics Committee Review
- Handling of Documents Requiring Signature: Indemnity, Financial Agreements, Confidentiality Agreements
- Registration with Hospital Management.

SOP 4
Local Management Requirements

Purpose

To ensure that any local administrative or management requirements are met.

Other Related Procedures

None in this manual. SOPs generated locally that apply are (complete details below):

Procedure

1. Who?

The Principal Investigator is responsible for ensuring that all local requirements are met.

2. When?

Before each clinical trial commences (i.e. before entry of the first patient into any trial-specific procedures), the appropriate local pre-trial requirements must be met.

Any requirements applying both during and after the completion of the trial must be met at all times.

3. How?

The Principal Investigator, or his or her designee, must establish from the local management details of existing regulations concerning clinical trials. If there are none, this should be documented and attached as an appendix to this SOP.

Any special requirements should be written up as an SOP (with checklist if appropriate) and carried out accordingly. At approximately yearly intervals the requirements should be reviewed and updated if there have been any changes in policy or requirements. The date of the review should be recorded by countersigning and dating the applicable SOPs at the time of review to state that they still apply.

Changes to local requirements that become known to members of the department before the review should be implemented according to local requirements and accompanied by the appropriate revision and re-issue of the SOPs affected.

SOP approved by: _____

Signature: _____ *Date:* _____

SOP 5
Review and Validation of the Protocol

Background

A protocol is defined as follows in the ICH GCP Guidelines: 'a document that describes the objective(s), design, methodology, statistical considerations, and organisation of a trial'. The guidelines also state that 'the protocol usually also gives the background and rationale for the trial'.

Section 6 of the guidelines provides a list of topics that protocols should generally include.

It is important that Investigators read and are familiar with the protocol. However, the Principal Investigator has additional responsibilities: firstly to check that the protocol is ethically acceptable (he/she must submit the study to the Ethics Committee and be able to justify the study on ethical grounds), and secondly to establish that the protocol is acceptable on clinical and practical grounds.

The protocol should be considered the backbone of the study. It contains the detailed 'why, what, when and how' of the study. In all the sections of any protocol, all definitions should be clear and not open to different interpretations. This is particularly important, for example, if there are particular grades of illness to be included or excluded, or if there are different diagnostic methods. Even quite common diagnoses should be described in detail. For example, to define hypertension, the upper and lower acceptable limits and the exact method of blood pressure measurement should be listed – whether it is measured sitting or lying, on the left or right side, and with which apparatus.

Most protocols written by or for Pharmaceutical Industry Sponsors are according to the details described in the ICH GCP Guidelines. Sponsors generally develop protocols according to their own SOPs which are based on these guidelines.

If the procedure is used to evaluate a draft copy of a protocol, it will help identify areas which may benefit from revision. If the protocol is the final version, the procedure can be used to assess whether the study is suitable for the department.

SOP 5
Review and Validation of the Protocol

Purpose

This SOP is designed to assist department staff in the checking of a protocol prepared by an external Sponsor, and is designed to enable adequate review of salient points. It may also be used as a guide for the preparation or review of site-generated protocols, or assisting an external Sponsor in writing a protocol.

Other Related Procedures

SOP 10: Ethics Committee
SOP 3: Study Files and Filing

Procedure

1. Who?

The Principal Investigator is responsible for ensuring both external and internal protocols have adequate review. Review will be carried out by individuals with the appropriate expertise: this should include, where appropriate and where required, a Co-Investigator together with a Study Site Co-ordinator and Study Nurse. If the Principal Investigator feels the department staff are inadequately qualified to make assessments as to the adequacy of any aspects of the trial, for example the statistical methods or design of the trial, an expert opinion should be sought.

2. When?

For trials where the protocol is generated externally, this procedure should be carried out as soon as is practical after the department receives a copy of the protocol. Feedback regarding the suitability of the protocol (for conduct in the department) should be given to the Sponsor at the earliest opportunity.

3. How?

In checking the protocol, remember that the ideal clinical situation is not always the ideal clinical trial situation, and most study protocols are a compromise between the two.

• The first piece of information to check is the **title**. What sort of a study is it, for what indication and with which investigational product?

SOP 5
Review and Validation of the Protocol

- The names of the **Investigators** and **other participants** (if fully identified/agreed at this stage) and the name of the **Sponsor** (if any) should appear somewhere on the protocol – usually on the title page or as an appendix.
- The protocol must describe the **aim** of the trial and present the rationale for doing it, together with a summary of the question to be addressed. The background to these points must be adequately referenced. Any therapeutic alternatives for the condition under study should also be summarised. The aim of the trial should be summarised in one or very few **primary objectives**.
- There must be a description of the general **design** of the trial – which phase it is, the randomisation method, design, blinding technique, and other bias reducing factors.
- The **ethical considerations** must be described including a description of the method of obtaining informed consent.
- **Subject selection** is a critical section of the protocol – here the demographics of the patient population to be studied, the (precisely defined) diagnosis, and the inclusion and exclusion criteria must be described.
- The **methods** section should lay out clearly what to do and when. This should include details about treatment and methods of evaluation.
- A **time schedule** for the trial must be included and justified. The duration of use of an investigational drug in humans is initially dictated by the number and duration of safety tests in animal experiments, and this must be taken into account.
- The **treatment** must also be described in detail. This should include: the name of the product, its presentation, administration, dose, concomitant medication, measures for safe handling and compliance monitoring, and details of the treatment for controls.
- How will the **efficacy and safety** of the treatments be assessed? This must be precisely specified with a description of the measurement and recording, the times of measurement, and any special analyses.
- How the **response** is to be **evaluated**, with the computation and calculation of effects, dealing with withdrawals and drop outs, and quality control methods, must be described.

Review and Validation of the Protocol

- Methods of recording **adverse events** and how to deal with complications, code breaking, reporting of adverse events: by whom, to whom, and how fast, should all be written in the protocol.
- There should also be a section about the practicalities of how the trial will be **monitored**, the specifications and instructions for deviations from the protocol, addresses and contact telephone numbers, and confidentiality problems, if any.
- There must also be a **statistical section** containing statistical assumptions and planned analytical methods, justification for the number of patients, level of significance, and the rules for termination and interim analysis, if necessary. The trial should be designed to have at least reasonable chance of meeting all the primary objectives and these should all be addressed in this section.
- Other sections might include:
  - The handling of records – such as the procedure for a patient list, and the CRFs
  - Financing, reporting, approvals, insurance/liability/indemnity etc.
  - A summary of the protocol
  - Appendix/Supplements – patient information leaflet, consent form, description of special procedures
  - References.
- In all the sections of the protocol, all definitions must be clear and not open to different interpretations.

Signing of the protocol

Only when the Principal Investigator has examined the protocol and agreed its suitability should it be signed and dated. If there are any outstanding problems or questions these should be discussed with the Sponsor before signing.

SOP approved by: _____

Signature: _____ *Date:* _____

SOP 5 – CHECKLIST
Review and Validation of the Protocol

Protocol Code: [   ]   Date of Protocol: [| | |]
                                                    dd mm yy

Abbreviated Title: _____

Sponsor Name: _____

	Yes	No	Comments (see end) (comment no.)
Is the protocol a draft version?	☐ *	☐ **	☐
*If yes, what is the draft number?	☐		
**If no, is it the final version?	☐	☐	

	Yes	No	Comments (see end) (comment no.)
Are there any amendments?	☐	☐	☐

If yes, how many? [ ]   Ensure these are kept with the protocol

Protocol/Study Number: [   ]

Title of study:

Who is Sponsor for the study? _____

	Yes	No	Comments (see end) (comment no.)
Has the Sponsor agreed to take on the responsibilities of the Sponsor as defined in the ICH Guidelines?	☐	☐	☐

Name of test medication: [   ]

SOP 5 – CHECKLIST
Review and Validation of the Protocol

	Yes	No	Comments (see end) (comment no.)
Is it a multi-centre trial?	☐	☐	☐
If yes, number of centres:	☐		

	Yes	No	Comments (see end) (comment no.)
Is there a flowchart for the study?	☐	☐	☐
Is there a summary for the study?	☐	☐	☐
Is the aim of the study adequately explained?	☐	☐	☐
Do the references supplied support the statements in the rationale?	☐	☐	☐

Ethical aspects	Yes	No	Comments (see end) (comment no.)
Is written informed consent required? If no, this must be adequately justified in the comments.	☐	☐	☐
Is the confidentiality of the patient adequately protected? If no, this must be adequately discussed in the comments.	☐	☐	☐
Will there be any payment to the subjects?	☐	☐	☐
May the study be published even if the study drug does not show an advantage over standard treatment?	☐	☐	☐
In randomised trials, is the available evidence for a difference between treatments under study adequate?	☐	☐	☐

SOP 5 – CHECKLIST
Review and Validation of the Protocol

Planned time schedule

Start of recruitment: ⊔⊔ month ⊔⊔ year

End of recruitment: ⊔⊔ month ⊔⊔ year

Last patient fully documented: ⊔⊔ month ⊔⊔ year

	Yes	No	Comments (see end) (comment no.)
Is the Principal Investigator satisfied that the length of treatment per patient is in accordance with the pre-clinical testing?	☐	☐	☐

Refer to Investigator's Brochure or Sponsor if required for toxicological data.

How long will each patient be followed up after treatment? ⊔⊔ days/weeks/months

Phase of the study   I   ☐

II   ☐

III   ☐

IV   ☐

SOP 5 – CHECKLIST
Review and Validation of the Protocol

Study Design

Randomisation (tick - ✓ - one)

Randomised: ☐

Non-randomised: ☐

Controls (tick - ✓ - one)   **Details** (tick - ✓ - at least one)

Comparator or control: ☐   reference drug: ☐ **Names**

No comparator: ☐   no treatment: ☐ **of reference**

placebo: ☐ **drugs**

Blinding (tick - ✓ - one)   **Details** (tick - ✓ - appropriate)

Open trial: ☐   Single blind: ☐

Blind trial: ☐   Double blind: ☐

Double dummy: ☐

Statistical Design (tick - ✓ - all appropriate)

Parallel group design: ☐

Crossover: ☐

Dose incrementation: ☐

Factorial: ☐

Matched Pairs: ☐

Sequential: ☐

Description of Aims (tick - ✓ - all appropriate)   **Details if 'Other'**

Efficacy and safety: ☐

Tolerability: ☐

Quality of life study: ☐

Cost–benefit study: ☐

Other (details): ☐

Selection of Study Population:

Comments
(see end)
(comment no.)

Inclusion Criteria

Too strict ☐

(Tick - ✓ - one) Too lenient ☐   ☐

Acceptable ☐

(Tick - ✓ - one) Clearly defined ☐   ☐

Ambiguous ☐

SOP 5 – CHECKLIST
Review and Validation of the Protocol

Exclusion Criteria

Comments
(see end)
(comment no.)

(Tick -✓- one)	Too strict: ☐	
	Too lenient: ☐	☐
	Acceptable: ☐	
(Tick -✓- one)	Clearly defined: ☐	☐
	Ambiguous: ☐	

	Yes	No	Comments (see end) (comment no.)
Will the study population be representative of a sufficiently wide patient population to enable the proposed number to be recruited in the allotted time?	☐	☐	☐

Is the description of the study drugs and their use acceptable . . . with regard to:

	Yes	No	Comments (see end) (comment no.)
Route of administration?	☐	☐	☐
Dose – amount and frequency?	☐	☐	☐
Concomitant medication?	☐	☐	☐
Any run-in, wash-out, or follow-up periods?	☐	☐	☐
Possible side effects and dose modification?	☐	☐	☐
Supply of study drug by Sponsor?	☐	☐	☐
Control group: acceptability of control treatment?	☐	☐	☐
Blinding?	☐	☐	☐

Efficacy Criteria

	Yes	No	Comments (see end) (comment no.)
Are the efficacy criteria clinically relevant and patient orientated? If no, this must be adequately discussed in the comments.	☐	☐	☐
Is there *one* principal criterion for assessment of treatment response? If no, this must be adequately discussed in the comments.	☐	☐	☐
Are the efficacy criteria clearly defined? If no, this must be adequately discussed in the comments.	☐	☐	☐
Are the methods of assessment of the efficacy criteria adequate and without biases? If no, this must be adequately discussed in the comments.	☐	☐	☐

SOP 5 – CHECKLIST
Review and Validation of the Protocol

Adverse Events	Yes	No	Comments (see end) (comment no.)
Is the procedure for reporting adverse events adequately detailed in the protocol?	☐	☐	☐
Are the methods for dose modification and treatment discontinuation adequately described?	☐	☐	☐

Evaluation	Yes	No	Comments (see end) (comment no.)
Are plans for evaluation of protocol violators clearly defined?	☐	☐	☐
Are methods for evaluating premature withdrawals adequately described?	☐	☐	☐
Are guidelines concerning the replacement of withdrawals clear?	☐	☐	☐

Statistics – specification and justification of:	Yes	No	Comments (see end) (comment no.)
Statistical hypotheses for the trial, including power and levels of significance	☐	☐	☐
Sample size	☐	☐	☐
Analysis	☐	☐	☐
Interim analyses or data inspections	☐	☐	☐

Have the following points been reviewed and found acceptable?	Yes	No	Comments (see end) (comment no.)
Data collection material (CRFs*, diary cards, Quality of Life questionnaire. If yes, specify which)	☐	☐	☐
Financing of the trial	☐	☐	☐
Indemnity/insurance and liability	☐	☐	☐
Patient information/consent form	☐	☐	☐
Descriptions of special procedures	☐	☐	☐
Appendices	☐	☐	☐
Monitoring of trial?	☐	☐	☐
Publishing agreement?	☐	☐	☐

*see checklist in SOP 7

SOP 5 – CHECKLIST
Review and Validation of the Protocol

Summarise the points that need further discussion with the Sponsor:

Discussed (Date)

1. _____   / /

2. _____   / /

3. _____   / /

4. _____   / /

5. _____   / /

6. _____   / /

	Yes	No	Comments (see end) (comment no.)
If final, has the Principal Investigator checked and signed the protocol?	☐	☐	☐

*If yes, date of signing   ⊔⊔ day   ⊔⊔ month   ⊔⊔ year

Signed by: _____

Checklist completed by: _____ *on* _____

(date)

SOP 5 – CHECKLIST
Review and Validation of the Protocol

<u>Comments</u> (Number the comments in the left-hand column)

SOP 6
Review of Protocol Amendments

Background

It may be necessary during the course of the study to make amendments to the protocol. For example, the inclusion criteria may prove to be too strict, thus making enrolment of patients difficult, or adverse events may occur which make an adjustment to the dose of the study medication necessary. An SOP specifying how such amendments are dealt with is, therefore, essential.

SOP 6
Review of Protocol Amendments

Purpose

To describe the procedure for reviewing any proposed changes to the protocol that may be introduced during the study.

Other Related Procedures

SOP 5: Review and Validation of the Protocol
SOP 10: Ethics Committee
SOP 3: Study Files and Filing

Procedure

1. Who?

The Principal Investigator must check all amendments before signing them and must ensure that all staff are informed of the amendment.

The individual responsible for the study must ensure that all staff are informed in a timely fashion.

2. When?

Staff should be made aware of the proposed amendment at the earliest opportunity. As soon as the amendment is available, the various actions detailed in 'How?' should be implemented. If the amendment removes from patients, or reduces, the likelihood of a hazard discovered during the course of the trial, it should be implemented immediately it is agreed.

3. How?

On determining the need for, or advantage that would obtain from, the introduction of an amendment to the protocol, all relevant parties should be consulted before the amendment is implemented. Where there is an external Sponsor, no amendment to the protocol may be implemented without the expressed agreement of the Sponsor.

On receiving an amendment from an external Sponsor, the Principal Investigator must review it in conjunction with the protocol. If in agreement with the amendment, it shall be signed. The Principal Investigator must then ensure that all staff are aware that an amendment to the protocol exists and are aware of its content.

SOP 6
Review of Protocol Amendments

Sponsors have different methods of producing amendments – sometimes it will be an additional page, sometimes the whole protocol will be rewritten as an amended version, especially if the amendment causes changes throughout the protocol. If the amendment is supplied as a loose leaf page, it is to be recommended that a hand-written comment is made at the appropriate part of the original protocol, to indicate the existence of the amendment. The amendment should be filed together with the protocol.

If the protocol is rewritten as a new version, one old version should be filed and endorsed to make it apparent to a prospective reader that it has been superseded and on what date. The remaining protocols should be returned to the Sponsor or destroyed. Do not destroy the old version before checking with the Sponsor. Be wary storing the old version, as this can lead to confusion if the wrong version is referred to during the trial.

The Ethics Committee must be informed of the amendment. Except where necessary to eliminate an immediate hazard, or when the change involves only logistical or administrative aspects of the trial, the amendment should not be implemented without documented approval from the Ethics Committee.

SOP approved by: _____

Signature: _____ *Date:* _____

SOP 6 – CHECKLIST
Review of Protocol Amendments

Protocol Code: [   ]   Date of Protocol: [| | |]
                                                  dd mm yy

Abbreviated Title: _____

Sponsor Name: _____

Summary of the reason for the amendment:

	Yes	No	Comments (see end) (comment no.)
Is protocol acceptable with the amendment? (If necessary complete a new checklist for protocol validation and indicate that you have done so in the comments)	☐	☐	☐
Does the amendment involve only logistical or administrative aspects or eliminate immediate hazard?	☐ *	☐	☐

* If no, Ethics Committee approval must be obtained before the amendment can be implemented.

What form does the amendment take?

Additional loose leaf   ☐

New, revised version of complete protocol   ☐

SOP 6 – CHECKLIST
Review of Protocol Amendments

	Yes	No	Comments (see end) (comment no.)
If loose leaf: has a note been made in the original protocol?	☐	☐	☐
If new version: has the old version been endorsed and filed and spare copies been returned to the Sponsor?	☐	☐	☐

	Yes	No	Comments (see end) (comment no.)
Has the amendment been approved and signed by the Principal Investigator?*	☐	☐	☐
Has the amendment been submitted to the Ethics Committee?	☐	☐	☐
**Has the amendment been approved by the Ethics Committee?	☐	☐	☐

*Date of signature: ⊔⊔ ⊔⊔ ⊔⊔
                     day   month   year

**Date approved: ⊔⊔ ⊔⊔ ⊔⊔
                     day   month   year

Checklist completed by: _____ *on* _____
(date)

SOP 6 – CHECKLIST
Review of Protocol Amendments

<u>Comments</u> (Number the comments in the left-hand column)

SOP 7
Case Report Form (CRF) Review

Background

Before the first patient is enrolled in the trial, the Sponsor must design and prepare the case report forms. At one of the centres in the trial, the Sponsor may ask that the CRF be checked, or request a complete dummy-run with a patient. Where there is no external Sponsor, case report forms must be designed and the preparation overseen by appropriate staff at the study site.

One aim is to detect weaknesses in a draft CRF that may be improved to make the finished forms as easy to complete as possible.

Another aim is to attempt to identify ambiguities, difficulties and possibly missing items in finalised CRFs before the CRF is used to collect 'real data'.

SOP 7
Case Report Form (CRF) Review

Purpose

To describe the procedure for reviewing and validating CRFs before the start of the trial.

Other Related Procedures

SOP 19: Case Report Form (CRF) Completion

Procedure

1. Who?

The CRF should generally be a stand-alone document, and sufficiently clear to an individual without specific knowledge of the trial.

Wherever possible, at least one member of the research team should check the CRFs. If an Investigator has been closely involved in designing and writing the protocol, it is better if he/she does not check the CRFs.

It is preferable that, of the individuals reviewing draft CRFs, at least one should be someone who will complete them during the trial.

2. When?

Review of a draft CRF should occur as soon as possible after receiving it. There can be a tight schedule in the weeks leading up to the start of the trial and postponements, because CRFs are not ready, can be significant.

From the time of making the final corrections to a CRF and having them returned from the printer most Sponsors need to allow a minimum of four weeks.

3. How?

During the first meeting(s) with the Monitor, or other representative of the Sponsor setting up the study, identify whether the centre will be involved in checking draft CRFs.

Where possible, try to complete the test CRF in a true-to-life situation, using real source documents when filling in the forms.

Where possible, compare the CRF with others from similar trials to highlight deficiencies.

Complete a CRF checklist.

If several staff are involved in testing the CRFs at the department, complete the CRFs independently and compare notes afterwards.

Inform the Sponsor of comments as soon as possible in writing.

SOP 7
Case Report Form (CRF) Review

If the CRF under review is a draft, request in writing that the Sponsor inform the individual responsible for the trial of a summary of the changes that will be made following the review. If the CRF under review is not a draft, request in writing that the Sponsor responds to the comments to the individual responsible for the trial.

SOP approved by: _____

Signature: _____ *Date:* _____

SOP 7 – CHECKLIST
Case Report Form (CRF) Review

Protocol Code: [   ]   Date of Protocol: | | | |
                                                  dd mm yy

Abbreviated Title: _____

Sponsor Name: _____

Are the following points included in the CRFs?	Yes (✔)	No (✔)	Comments (see end) (comment no.)
Some kind of trial identification?	☐	☐	☐
Patient identification code/initials? (The patient's full name should **not** appear on the CRF)	☐	☐	☐
Demographic data on each patient?	☐	☐	☐
Diagnosis of the patient?	☐	☐	☐
Inclusion and exclusion criteria?	☐	☐	☐
Administration of the study medication?	☐	☐	☐
Recording of concomitant medications?	☐	☐	☐
Recording of efficacy parameters?	☐	☐	☐
Recording of adverse events?	☐	☐	☐
Reasons for withdrawal?	☐	☐	☐

Comment on the following points:	Yes (✔)	No (✔)	Comments (see end) (comment no.)
Are the instructions for completing the CRFs clear?	☐	☐	☐
Are the forms well laid out?	☐	☐	☐
Is the order of the questions logical?	☐	☐	☐
Do you find the forms too detailed?	☐	☐	☐
Not detailed enough?	☐	☐	☐
Do you ever need to complete the same data twice?	☐	☐	☐
Do you have difficulty understanding any of the questions, e.g. knowing whether to tick 'yes' or 'no'?	☐	☐	☐

SOP 7 – CHECKLIST
Case Report Form (CRF) Review

Are there any abbreviations or terms which you did not immediately understand? ☐ ☐ ☐

Is it always clear what needs to be completed and when? ☐ ☐ ☐

Do you need to refer to the protocol or Investigator's Brochure to complete the form? ☐ ☐ ☐

For written responses – is there enough space to write your answer? ☐ ☐ ☐

Which points need raising with the Sponsor?

_____

_____

_____

_____

Are CRFs: Draft? ☐   or Final? ☐

Date important items above raised with Sponsor: ⊔⊔ ⊔⊔ ⊔⊔   By: _____
                                       day month year

CRFs accepted on: ⊔⊔ ⊔⊔ ⊔⊔   By: _____
                        day month year

Checklist completed by: _____ _on_ _____
                                                       (date)

SOP 7 – CHECKLIST
Case Report Form (CRF) Review

Comments (Number the comments in the left-hand column)

SOP 8
Investigator's Brochure

Background

The Investigator's Brochure or the equivalent information must be supplied by the Sponsor to each study centre taking part in a clinical trial. It contains all the relevant information known prior to the onset of a clinical trial including chemical and pharmaceutical data, toxicological, pharmacokinetics and pharmacodynamic data in animals and the results of earlier clinical trials. There should be adequate data to justify the nature, scale and duration of the proposed trial.

It may be the case that for Phase IV studies no Investigator's Brochure is supplied because the drug is already registered with the authorities and the summary of product characteristics will be used instead.

SOP 8
Investigator's Brochure

Purpose

To describe the procedures associated with the Investigator's Brochure.

Other Related Procedures

SOP 13: Pre-study Monitoring Visits
SOP 10: Ethics Committee
SOP 3: Study Files and Filing

Procedure

1. Who?

The Principal Investigator and all Investigators working on the study.

2. When?

Before agreeing to act as an Investigator in a study all Investigators must have read and be familiar with the Investigator's Brochure.

3. How?

Check with the Sponsor whether an Investigator's Brochure will be provided. For all studies with investigational products, i.e. not yet registered, an Investigator's Brochure should be provided.

All Investigators must know where the Investigator's Brochure is kept.

Frequently two copies of the Investigator's Brochure will be supplied to a centre, one copy remains in the department, the other copy is submitted to the Ethics Committee with the other documents.

If any new information arises during the trial, the Monitor should supply the department with an update or a revised version of the Investigator's Brochure. The Principal Investigator must ensure that all Investigators are familiar with the updated Investigator's Brochure.

One way for all Investigators to become familiar with the Investigator's Brochure is for each Investigator to prepare a short talk for each section of the brochure.

Remember that the Investigator's Brochure contains highly confidential data and only people directly involved in the study should have access to the information.

SOP approved by: _____

Signature: _____ *Date:* _____

SOP 8 – CHECKLIST
Investigator's Brochure

Protocol Code: [   ]   Date of Protocol: | | | |
                                                      dd mm yy

Abbreviated Title: _____

Sponsor Name: _____

Is an Investigator's Brochure available?   Yes ☐

                                                   No   ☐

If no, what alternative is available?

_____

If yes, give details.

    Title of Investigator's Brochure _____

_____

    Date of version _____

If Investigator's Brochure has individual number, what is it? _____

Who else holds Investigator's Brochure at the centre (e.g. Pharmacy)? _____

_____

Is a separate copy of the Investigator's Brochure to be provided for the Ethics Committee?

_____

SOP 9
Estimation of Patient Numbers

Background

In the days before GCP, clinical trials were often planned and performed with such small sample sizes that no reliable conclusions could be drawn. From a purely ethical standpoint this is unacceptable.

In Section 6 of the ICH GCP Guidelines there is a section on the content of the trial protocol, including Section 6.9 on Statistics. Here it states that the protocol should contain 'the number of patients planned to be enrolled ... Reason for choice of sample size, including reflections on (or calculations of) the power of the trial and clinical justification'. In other words, in a comparative trial, the number of patients in each sample group must be calculated or justified.

This may be done by estimating the percentage of successful treatments in each of the treatment groups at the end of the trial. Limits must also be set, firstly as to the acceptable risk of obtaining a false positive result (one treatment appears to be better than the other when it isn't), and secondly, the acceptable risk of obtaining a false negative result (the two treatments appear to have the same efficacy, when in fact one is better than the other). These are known as the alpha and beta error, respectively. When all these figures are put into the right equation, you can calculate the number of subjects required for the study.

All GCP standard studies should now be performed with adequate patient numbers and thus have the potential of detecting a real difference between two treatments.

Which brings us to the next problem of actually finding the calculated number of patients to fulfil the study requirements – this is one of the major stumbling blocks in clinical research. Accurate estimation of patient numbers by Investigators at the study site is a vital stage in the planning of a clinical study. In the past, accurate estimates were the exception rather than the rule.

This procedure is designed to give you some pointers as to how you can best estimate the size of potential patient populations.

SOP 9
Estimation of Patient Numbers

Purpose

To provide a standard, reliable procedure for the estimation of the number of patients that can be enrolled in a trial.

Other Related Procedures

SOP 13: Pre-study Monitoring Visits
SOP 14: Patient Recruitment and Intention to Enrol

Procedure

1. Who?

The statistician will have calculated the required sample size.

The procedure for estimating patient numbers should be co-ordinated by the Principal Investigator or his/her designee, but may involve all doctors in the department and possibly, if the study centre is a referral department, external departments who refer cases to your department.

2. When?

The likely patient numbers for the department should normally be estimated after the first contact with your department by the Sponsor of the study.

It may be the case that during the study recruitment is not as good as was estimated and a re-estimation is necessary.

3. How?

The statistical section of the protocol should contain details of how the patient numbers were calculated. The parameters for the study should be checked to ensure they are clinically realistic, for example percentage drop out rate, expected response rate etc. (See SOP 5: Review and Validation of the Protocol.)

A discussion with the Sponsor (or Monitor) about the inclusion and exclusion criteria for the trial is essential. Depending on how strict the criteria are, a large proportion of what you believe to be suitable patients may be excluded from the study at this stage.

Exactly how you then estimate the number of potential patients will to an extent depend on the protocol. Possibilities are:

SOP 9
Estimation of Patient Numbers

- Examination of medical records and patient notes

For chronic conditions, the records can be checked through to find all patients with the appropriate diagnosis for the study who also satisfy the inclusion and exclusion criteria. From this number, allowance must be made for patients who are unable or unwilling to participate in the study. There are, however, a multitude of factors to take into consideration, including design of the trial, and even time of year, e.g. for allergic conditions.

- Assessment of patients visiting clinic during the pre-study period

If it is an acute condition, for example a shock therapy, either the records of patients coming to the clinic over the last number of months or years can be checked, or a pilot run can be done during the pre-study period, if there is enough time. This method can only be used for conditions which are quite common.

- Examination of previous clinical trials

If trials have been done in the clinic before for the particular indication, recruitment rates can be used as a guide. Care should be taken to ensure that the inclusion and exclusion criteria are comparable.

- Assessment of any concurrently running studies

This may be an obvious point, but there should be no overlap in the patient populations because this would reduce potential numbers. (Another point to raise here – if there are too many studies going on at once, recruitment will suffer because of overwork and lack of time!)

The numbers estimated will be used to calculate recruitment goals for the department (see SOP 14: Patient Recruitment and Intention to Enrol).

SOP approved by: _____

Signature: _____ *Date:* _____

SOP 9 – CHECKLIST
Estimation of Patient Numbers

Protocol Code: [_____]   Date of Protocol: |_|_|_|
                                              dd mm yy

Abbreviated Title: _____

Sponsor Name: _____

Which condition is under investigation? _____

	Yes	No	Comments (see end) (comment no.)
Is it a special sub-group of patients?	☐	☐	☐

	Yes	No	Comments (see end) (comment no.)
Do you see any problem with the inclusion and exclusion criteria?	☐	☐	☐

	Yes	No	Comments (see end) (comment no.)
Is the condition acute?	☐	☐	☐
Is the condition chronic or recurring?	☐	☐	☐
Do you see any problems with the protocol regarding reluctance of patients to give their consent?	☐	☐	☐

Method of estimating patient numbers		Number estimated	Comments (see end) (comment no.)
Examination of records and patient notes	☐	___	☐
Assessment during pre-study period	☐	___	☐
Recruitment rates in previous studies	☐	___	☐

SOP 9 – CHECKLIST
Estimation of Patient Numbers

		Number estimated	Comments (see end) (comment no.)
Concurrent studies – overlapping populations	☐	___	☐
Other: _____	☐	___	☐
In clinic only	☐	___	☐
Contacting referral centres	☐	___	☐

A more precise study-specific checklist may be drawn up. For example: how many patients with diagnosis X were treated at (clinic) in the last three months? Of these, how many received treatment and responded as defined in the protocol?

It may be possible that if the numbers obtained from the first estimates are too low, the protocol may be reassessed, particularly with reference to the inclusion and exclusion criteria. Which parameter(s) would you suggest to alter?

1. _____

2. _____

3. _____

4. _____

Checklist completed by: _____ *on* _____
(date)

SOP 9 – CHECKLIST
Estimation of Patient Numbers

__Comments__ (Number the comments in the left-hand column)

SOP 10
Ethics Committee

Background

Ethical approval of clinical trials is one of the main themes of the Declaration of Helsinki: 'The design and performance of each experimental procedure involving human subjects should be clearly formulated in an experimental protocol which should be transmitted for consideration, comment and guidance to a specially appointed committee independent of the Investigator and the Sponsor provided that this independent committee is in conformity with the laws and regulations of the country in which the research experiment is performed.'

The division of the responsibilities between the Investigator and the Sponsor concerning notification to the Ethics Committee must be arranged at the study planning phase.

The Ethics Committee will examine and consider the following points:

- The suitability of the Investigator for the proposed trial, including their qualifications, experience, supporting staff, and available facilities.
- The data available on the drug (or device) under study.
- The suitability of the protocol, including the objectives of the study, the potential for reaching sound conclusions with the smallest possible exposure of subjects, and a weighing up of the possible risks and inconveniences with possible benefits to the patient and others.
- The suitability of the patient information and consent forms and procedure.
- The means of recruitment.
- The provision for compensation and/or treatment in the case of injury or death of a subject if attributable to a clinical trial, and any insurance or indemnity to cover the liability of the Investigator and Sponsor.
- The extent to which Investigators and subjects may be rewarded and/or compensated for participation.

SOP 10
Ethics Committee

Purpose

To describe your duties concerning ethical approval of the clinical study by an Ethics Committee.

Other Related Procedures

SOP 6: Review of Protocol Amendments
SOP 15: Obtaining Personal Written Informed Consent
SOP 22: Adverse Event and Serious Adverse Event Reporting
SOP 3: Study Files and Filing
SOP 11: Indemnity, Compensation and Insurance

Procedure

1. Who?

If it has been arranged that the Sponsor submits the study for Ethics Committee approval, the Principal Investigator must, prior to the submission, agree to the informed consent procedure, and after submission, ensure that Ethics Committee approval has been obtained (request a copy of the letter of approval and file this in the Study File).

If the responsibility lies with the Investigator, he or she should work according to this procedure. The Sponsor will often provide any necessary administrative or financial support – again these details must be agreed at the planning stage of the study. The Investigator may designate a member of staff to prepare the submission but should take responsibility for it by signing it off.

2. When?

At the earliest opportunity the Principal Investigator must check when the Ethics Committee holds its meetings. If it does not meet very often this can delay the start of the trial. He/she should also check the normal response time.

Written approval must obviously be obtained before the first patient is enrolled in the study.

During the trial, contact must be maintained with the Ethics Committee, and the Committee must be notified of the end of the trial.

SOP 10
Ethics Committee

3. How?

<u>Before Study Start</u>

In multi-centre studies the submission may have to be co-ordinated if more than one centre is using the same Ethics Committee.

It may be necessary that each centre must independently obtain Ethics Committee approval, or that one central Ethics Committee approves the trial for all centres.

The required number of copies of the trial protocol and all annexes must be submitted to the Ethics Committee, together with the methods and material to be used in obtaining and documenting informed consent of the subjects and a covering letter (see Procedure 3/3, 'Documentation').

In non-English-speaking countries, if appropriate, check whether documents in English are acceptable for the Ethics Committee. Translations may be required, at least of the protocol summary.

The patient's informed consent forms must anyway be in a language that the patient can understand.

The curriculum vitae or qualifications of all Investigators and Co-Investigators involved in the trial should be submitted to the Ethics Committee.

If, before approval of the study, the Ethics Committee makes any recommendations for improvement, these should be acted upon immediately by the Principal Investigator or a designated individual.

<u>During the Study</u>

If there are any protocol amendments or serious or unexpected adverse events which are likely to affect the safety of the subjects or the conduct of the trial the Ethics Committee must be informed. The Committee should be asked for its opinion if a re-evaluation of the ethical aspects of the trial appears to be called for.

The Ethics Committee may require interim or periodic reports of the trial.

<u>End of Study</u>

You must inform the Ethics Committee that the trial has ended.

4. Documentation

Covering letter

The letter submitted to the Ethics Committee should contain a request to review the protocol, with a summary of the rationale behind the study and the plans for the protection of the subjects. Potential ethical 'problem areas', for example necessity of screening tests involving very invasive procedures, e.g. biopsy, should be itemised and ethically justified.

The situation regarding insurance and indemnity should also be clarified in the letter, together with the situation regarding Investigator and any relevant subject payments if these items are inadequately explained elsewhere in the application.

- The opinion of the Ethics Committee should contain: an identification of the trial, the documents studied and the date of review, together with its opinion and advice.

All documentation relating to the Ethics Committee must be filed in the Study File and copies sent to the Sponsor.

SOP approved by: _____

Signature: _____ *Date:* _____

SOP 10 – CHECKLIST
Ethics Committee

Protocol Code: [   ]   Date of Protocol: [| | |]
                                                      dd mm yy

Abbreviated Title: _____

Sponsor Name: _____

The following checklist is intended for studies where the Principal Investigator submits the study for Ethics Committee approval. It should be completed and updated at appropriate intervals, at least once yearly. It can be kept in your SOP file as a reference for future studies.

	Yes	**No**	**Comments** (see end) (comment no.)
Will the study be assessed by a central Ethics Committee?	☐ *	☐	☐
*If yes, do you also require the approval of the hospital/health authority Ethics Committee?	☐	☐	☐

If a central Ethics Committee will approve the study, and not the local Ethics Committee, obtain a copy of the letter of the central approval for the Study File.

Name and address of chairperson of Ethics Committee:

Name   Dr/Mr/Ms _____   _____
                          (Forename)   (Surname)

Address   _____

                 _____

                 _____

When does the Ethics Committee sit?   **Yes**

On request   ☐

At regular intervals: monthly   ☐

                               bimonthly   ☐

                               quarterly   ☐

Other: _____

What is the normal response time? [   ] days

How many copies of the protocol are required? [   ]

How many copies of the patient information and consent are required? [   ]

SOP 10 – CHECKLIST
Ethics Committee

	Yes	No	Comments (see end) (comment no.)
Are there any other special requirements regarding the documents for submission?	☐ *	☐	☐
Are documents in English acceptable?	☐	☐	☐

*If yes, please give details below:

```
┌─────────────────────────────────────────────────────────────────┐
│                                                                   │
│                                                                   │
│                                                                   │
│                                                                   │
└─────────────────────────────────────────────────────────────────┘
```

For the study _____ :

	Yes	No	Comments (see end) (comment no.)
Has the protocol been checked by the Principal Investigator for its ethical content? (See separate checklist in SOP 5)	☐	☐	☐
Has a corresponding covering letter been written for the submission?	☐	☐	☐
When is the planned submission to the Ethics Committee?	⊔⊔ day	⊔⊔ month	⊔⊔ year

Documents submitted:	Yes	Number of copies	No	Not required
Protocol	☐	___	☐	☐
Protocol summary	☐	___	☐	☐
Patient information and consent form	☐	___	☐	☐
CVs of all Investigators	☐	___	☐	☐
Copy of insurance policy	☐	___	☐	☐
Investigator's Brochure	☐	___	☐	☐
Other: _____ (e.g. Case Report Forms)	☐	___	☐	☐

	Yes	No	Comments (see end) (comment no.)
Was approval of the study obtained?	☐ *	☐ **	☐

SOP 10 – CHECKLIST
Ethics Committee

*If yes,

- When was the Ethics Committee approval obtained?

　　　⊔⊔　　⊔⊔　　⊔⊔
　　　day　　month　　year

	Yes	No	Comments (see end) (comment no.)
• Has a letter of approval been obtained and filed?	☐	☐	☐

**If no, on what grounds was the submission refused?

```



```

	Yes	No	Comments (see end) (comment no.)
• Are any modifications necessary to then obtain approval?	☐ #	☐	☐

#If yes, give details here:

```



```

and give details below when Ethics Committee approval is given.

- Date approval obtained

　　　⊔⊔　　⊔⊔　　⊔⊔
　　　day　　month　　year

	Yes	No	Comments (see end) (comment no.)
• Has a letter of approval been obtained and filed?	☐	☐	☐

Checklist completed by: _____ *on* _____
　　　　　　　　　　　　　　　　　　　　　　　　　(date)

SOP 10 – CHECKLIST
Ethics Committee

Comments (Number the comments in the left-hand column)

SOP 11
Indemnity, Compensation and Insurance

Background

Clinical trials are experiments involving human subjects. By their nature, therefore, they often involve unproven procedures, devices or drugs under research. The evaluation of the procedure, device or drug in question may also lead the subject to be exposed to non-experimental procedures that carry more than a negligible risk. Such exposure to risk may be over and above that which the subject would incur under normal clinical conditions.

There are two distinct categories of subjects who participate in clinical trials: a) those who participate with no intended benefit to health (irrespective of the treatment allocated); b) those who take part in the knowledge that benefit may accrue from at least one of the treatments in the trial. The former are mostly so-called 'healthy volunteers', the latter are generally patient volunteers. The arrangements for ensuring adequate compensation in the event of injury are broadly similar in the two groups, but are likely to differ from country to country. For example, some countries offer 'no-fault' compensation in which payment will be offered from a fund without the need to establish 'blame'. Many trials involving healthy volunteers are conducted by Contract Research Organisations, and these generally have insurances to provide compensation for injury arising from participation in trials without the need to establish fault.

In the event of injury occurring as a result of participation in a clinical trial, a subject may desire compensation and seek to obtain this by legal action or otherwise. The parties who might be considered responsible for the well-being of the subject in the clinical trial are: the Sponsor or any of the Sponsor's agents, the Investigator, the Investigator's employer, the Investigator's Co-Investigators, the Investigator's other staff. This procedure sets out the means by which the Investigator should ensure adequate protection for subjects, him or herself, his or her employers and staff.

SOP 11

Indemnity, Compensation and Insurance

Purpose

To describe the procedure for ensuring that adequate financial compensation is available to subjects in the event of injury incurred in a clinical trial conducted at the department. To describe the procedure for ensuring adequate safeguarding of the Investigator, the Investigator's employer and other staff involved at the trial site in the event of a claim for compensation by a subject participating in a clinical trial.

Other Related Procedures

SOP 4: Local Management Requirements
SOP 22: Adverse Event and Serious Adverse Event Reporting

Procedure

1. Who?

The Investigator or study responsible individual is responsible for ensuring the necessary arrangements are in place and that the appropriate documents are signed by the appropriate individuals.

The Investigator must assume ultimate responsibility.

The Investigator and all staff at the department participating in the clinical trial are responsible for ensuring adherence to the study protocol, for ensuring documentation of deviations that do occur, and for ensuring appropriate communication to relevant parties in a timely manner when deviations occur.

The Investigator and all staff at the department participating in the clinical trial are responsible for communicating serious adverse events to relevant parties in a timely manner when they occur.

The Investigator is responsible for making information available to relevant parties in the event that this is required.

2. When?

All appropriate arrangements, documents and signatures should be obtained prior to any subject being exposed to any possible risk associated with the trial, preferably before the submission to the Ethics Committee is made.

Before each subject consents to participate in the trial, he or she must be informed that compensation will be available in the event of injury.

SOP 11

Indemnity, Compensation and Insurance

In the event of injury, or of a claim for injury, the subject will be informed that compensation can be sought, and provided with written details of how to make a claim. At the earliest opportunity in such a case, any external Sponsor, any relevant employer and other relevant parties will be informed.

3. How?

- The protocol must be read carefully to ensure adequate understanding of the clinical trial and the procedures involved.
- For a trial of a pharmaceutical agent, the safety of and experience with the drug must be considered (e.g. consult the Investigator's Brochure, or equivalent information).
- Any insurance arrangements, or similar, that are not specific to the trial but to individuals involved or the department as a whole must be current. Neither the trial nor the responsibilities of individuals involved in the trial should fall outside any terms of such arrangements. This should be checked if there is any uncertainty, and, where applicable, the scope of the arrangements be broadened if the trial is to be conducted. (Examples: Do doctors involved with the trial carry insurance such as that offered in the UK by the Medical Defence Union and others? Does the department carry a blanket insurance policy? If this trial is of a type not done previously at the department, or if different methods or staff will be used, are the terms adequate?)
- Where the terms of any such insurances make stipulations concerning general standards within the department (of equipment, training etc.), these must be met to ensure validity of the insurance.
- Where there is an external Sponsor, local management may require the signing of an indemnity. This should take a form explicitly approved by local management. If there is disparity between the form of words proposed by local management and that proposed by the Sponsor, the trial should not proceed until agreement is reached.
- Documents signed on behalf of the local management may be signed only by individuals authorised to do so.
- To comply with ICH GCP Guidelines, potential trial subjects must be informed in writing that compensation for injury will be available (e.g. in the patient information leaflet). In the event of injury, the Investigator must give the subject access to information about the procedures for compensation.

SOP 11
Indemnity, Compensation and Insurance

- If there are stipulations upon the subject that might affect the financial compensation for participation (such as in a healthy volunteer study), it should be clear in the information provided that compensation for injury is unaffected by them.
- The protocol should be adhered to; any deviations should be clearly documented.
- Adverse events must be elicited and recorded in accordance with the protocol.
- Serious adverse events must be identified and reported in accordance with the protocol and communicated to appropriate Sponsors and the Ethics Committee where applicable.
- The highest standards of medical practice must be followed by all doctors participating in the trial. The highest standards of healthcare must be followed by other staff involved with participating subjects.
- In the event of a subject suffering injury or claiming that injury has been suffered, the Investigator must make details of the procedure for applying for compensation available to the subject or the subject's representative. At the earliest opportunity the Investigator must inform local management and any external Sponsor of the likelihood of a claim, and provide information that is reasonably requested.

SOP approved by: _____

Signature: _____ *Date:* _____

SOP 11 – CHECKLIST
Indemnity, Compensation and Insurance

Protocol Code: [   ]   Date of Protocol: | | | |
                                                        dd mm yy

Abbreviated Title: _____

Sponsor Name: _____

Protocol

Does the trial involve patients, methods or procedures different from
those routinely used in the department?   **Yes/No**

Details if yes _____

Are there implications for any standing insurances?   **Yes/No**

Details if yes _____

Documentation

Which staff have insurance of any sort for their participation in the trial?

(Include personal insurances, professional insurances, insurance policies covering the
department as a whole)

Name	Details of Insurance

Are all standing insurances current and valid for this trial?   **Yes/No**

If no, what actions are to be taken? _____

Is indemnification required from an external Sponsor?   **Yes/No**

Is a standard form of words, known to be acceptable to local management,
also acceptable to the Sponsor?   **Yes/No**

If no, what actions are to be taken to ensure adequate indemnification of relevant parties
at the study site?

Who may sign the indemnity on behalf of local management?

SOP 11 – CHECKLIST
Indemnity, Compensation and Insurance

Information for Subjects

Does or will the subject information leaflet contain explicit wording to
convey the fact that compensation will be available in the event of injury?   **Yes/No**

If yes, give the (agreed) wording here. If no, explain, and give details of the intentions.

_____

In the event of injury or a claim for injury, what actions will be taken by the Investigator?

_____

_____

Serious Adverse Events

What will be the procedure for reporting serious events? Give details of standard forms,
timelines, parties to whom reports will be made.

_____

_____

_____

Checklist completed by: _____ _on_ _____
                                                              (date)

SOP 12
Laboratory

Background

Most clinical trials of pharmaceuticals require the taking of human samples for laboratory testing; the testing itself may occur at the study site or remotely at a 'central laboratory'. This is the common term given to laboratories that handle analysis and reporting of samples from a diversity of centres. Study site laboratories are usually those attached to a hospital. Central laboratories are often independent businesses, but can be a laboratory at a study site.

Procedures for the handling of samples for local processing will generally need to vary slightly for those sent for external testing, but the handling of reports will generally be the same.

SOP 12
Laboratory

Purpose

To describe the procedure for the general management of human trial samples and the resulting reports.

Other Related Procedures

SOP 5: Review and Validation of the Protocol

Procedure

1. Who?

The Investigator or individual(s) designated for the taking of samples: blood, urine etc. is responsible for ensuring the appropriate taking, handling, initial processing (such as centrifugation) and despatch of samples to the laboratory for analysis.

The Investigator must assume ultimate responsibility.

The study responsible individual must ensure that reports are dealt with appropriately in respect of the speed with which they are reviewed, that they are brought to the attention of the correct individual(s) and that appropriate information is provided to any external Sponsor as required.

2. When?

As early as possible, discussion should commence concerning the laboratories to be involved with the analysis of samples. The laboratories to be used should be agreed, in principle at least, before submission of the protocol to the Ethics Committee. Responsibility for supply of necessary materials should also be established early on to enable proper account to be taken in preparation of costings.

Before the entry of the first patient in the study, any instructions concerning the handling of samples must be established and any necessary training given.

Samples should be taken as per timings implied in the protocol.

Reports received must be reviewed at the earliest opportunity after arrival in the department, at least by the study responsible person. Review by an individual competent to act on the results should be ensured in line with good medical practice or the protocol if this requires speedier review.

Other doctors involved in the care of subjects participating in the trial should be notified of findings from laboratory reports as appropriate.

SOP 12
Laboratory

If appropriate, reports, or actions resulting from reports, should be notified to any external Sponsor in conformance with instructions provided.

3. How?

- Whether the trial involves samples for laboratory analysis must be established.
- The laboratory (if any) to be used must be identified and documented.
- Procedures for the taking, handling, initial processing within the department and despatch should be established and documented.
- The materials required should be identified and the responsibility for their supply be established.
- Any procedures that are not usual practice for the department should be documented and the documentation be readily available to all individuals involved with the samples or reports. Any possible difficulties that might arise in adhering to the procedures should be documented and communicated to the external Sponsor where applicable.
- Any training needs should be identified and the necessary training given (e.g. phlebotomy refresher course, slide preparation etc.).
- Staff dealing with samples in whatever capacity should be identified. This should include those considered 'qualified' (able) to take samples and contact names, telephone numbers and positions of relevant individuals at the appropriate laboratories.
- Staff should assist, as required, an external Sponsor to identify and liaise with appropriate individuals at local (on-site) laboratories. Such assistance should also extend to facilitating the appropriation of relevant documentation. This should include appropriate reference ranges, but may also include documents pertaining to Quality Assurance procedures in place within the laboratories.
- Where possible, samples should be taken according to requirements of the protocol. Deviations from the protocol should be documented with reasons for non-compliance.
- Non-adherence to specified procedures that might impact on results should be documented and made known to the study responsible individual, any individual reviewing the resulting report and the Sponsor.

SOP 12
Laboratory

- Laboratory reports should be brought to the attention of appropriate individuals at the earliest opportunity. The study responsible individual must ensure that reports are reviewed by individuals competent to do so.
- A standard practice for documenting the review of reports should be followed. For example, comments may be added to indicate the clinical significance of results and actions recommended; reports may be signed and dated by competent individuals. The aim should be to assure any external reviewer that the report has been adequately reviewed and appropriate actions taken.
- Reports, or duplicates of reports, should be maintained in an appropriate way to meet with local management requirements and those, where reasonable, of any external Sponsor. Above all, confidentiality of subjects to whom reports relate must be ensured.
- The subject's family doctor, where appropriate, and other doctors involved in the care of the individual as necessary should be notified of findings from laboratory reports.

SOP approved by: _____

Signature: _____ *Date:* _____

SOP 12 – CHECKLIST
Laboratory

Protocol Code: [_____]   Date of Protocol: |__|__|__|

　　　　　　　　　　　　　　　　　　　　　　　dd mm yy

Abbreviated Title: _____

Sponsor Name: _____

What is Required?

What samples are required for the trial?　Blood:　Whole blood　☐

　　　　　　　　　　　　　　　　　　　　　　Separated serum　☐

　　　　　　　　　　　　　　　　　　　　　　Separated plasma　☐

　　　　　　　　　　　　　Urine:　　　　　　　　　　　☐

　　　　　　　　　　　　　Other (specify):　　　　　　　☐

　　　　　　　　　　　　　　　　　　　　　　_____

　　　　　　　　　　　　　　　　　　　　　　_____

Where will Analysis be Carried Out?

Type of sample	Analysis, e.g. biochemistry, haematology etc.	Laboratory name	Non-routine external lab? Yes/No	Who will supply materials?	Contact name

Do any samples require freezing?　　　　　　　　　　　　　　**Yes/No**

If yes, give details: _____

For freezer samples ensure labels provided will be permanent　　**NA/Yes**

Documentation

For samples needing non-routine handling, and all samples analysed at non-routine external laboratories, documentation of procedure is required.

SOP 12 – CHECKLIST
Laboratory

Documentation required	Date obtained	Training needed? (Initials)*	Date given

*Put initials of staff for whom training is required. Also add here training needed for new staff for routine sampling.

Reference ranges required		

Procedure for Review of Reports

Who is responsible for handling/collating reports? _____

Who may review and sign off which reports?

Name	Type of Report
_____	_____
_____	_____
_____	_____
_____	_____

Detail of procedure for annotating received reports (e.g. 'Normal', Not Clinically Significant/NCS, Related to disease under study etc., signature of reviewer, date)

_____

_____

_____

Where will reports be filed/placed? (e.g. in case notes, CRFs): _____

Checklist completed by: _____ *Date:* _____

SOP 13
Pre-study Monitoring Visits

Background

There will be at least one Monitor (or CRA) assigned by the Sponsor to monitor the study. Monitors are often biological science graduates, sometimes medical doctors, sometimes with nursing qualifications. There is as yet no standard qualification required for Monitors of clinical trials. The Monitor's activities may range from visiting study centres (the activities which you will see), to designing the study and writing the protocol, to training staff at the department and subsequently writing the study report.

It is the responsibility of the study Monitor to visit the Investigator and the study site before, during and at the end of a clinical trial.

The Monitor will be working to the Sponsor's SOPs and there may be more than one pre-study visit planned to each centre. Exactly how many visits will vary from Sponsor to Sponsor and from study to study.

From the Sponsor's side there are several aims of the pre-study visits. These include:

- to introduce the study to the Investigator and their team.
- to ensure that the Investigator and their team have enough time, interest and experience to perform the study to the standard required.
- to assess the facilities and meet all individuals that might have some involvement with the trial, including those in other departments.

It is also an opportunity for the Investigator to assess both the Sponsor and the study.

In multi-centre studies there may be an Investigators' meeting planned. An Investigator (or delegated representative) from each centre should attend. The aim of the Investigators' meeting is to ensure a unified approach to the study protocol and documentation. Any outstanding or controversial points can be discussed.

SOP 13
Pre-study Monitoring Visits

Purpose

The objective of this procedure is to describe the probable procedure for site staff to follow for visits by the Monitor before official study start, i.e. before recruitment of the first patient. Included in this procedure are visits made by all representatives of the Sponsor to the study centre.

Other Related Procedures

SOP 5: Review and Validation of the Protocol
SOP 3: Study Files and Filing
SOP 2: Study Team: Definition of Responsibilities
SOP 14: Patient Recruitment and Intention to Enrol

Procedure

1. Who?

Who is present will depend on the stage of the study. For the initial pre-study visit, only the Principal Investigator need be present. The Principal Investigator must be present for at least part of at least one pre-trial meeting.

There is normally a study initiation meeting (or meetings) arranged to inform the entire study staff about the study and documentation – here, as many as possible of the staff who will be involved in the study should attend, i.e. the Principal Investigator, Sub-Investigators, the Study Site Co-ordinator (if there is one), pharmacist, and any nursing, laboratory, technical or administrative staff.

2. When?

Before enrollment of the first patient, but the exact schedule will vary.

3. How?

- At pre-study meetings (usually the initial meeting) the main task is for the Principal Investigator and/or other staff to assess acceptability and feasibility of the study protocol (see SOP 5: Review and Validation of the Protocol and associated checklist).
- Other salient points include discussion and agreement about division of the responsibilities according to GCP. For example, submission to the Ethics Committee, insurance arrangements, publication agreements and financial agreements.
- The scope of the trial should also be discussed so that site staff can estimate the requirements of the study regarding staff, facilities, financing etc.
- Written notes should be made for all meetings and kept in the Study File.

SOP 13
Pre-study Monitoring Visits

- In the course of the pre-study visits Sponsors require to be provided with the following documentation:
  - Curriculum vitae of the Principal Investigator and Sub-Investigators.
  - Signed copy of protocol plus any amendments.
  - List of laboratory reference ranges and details of Quality Control/Quality Assurance Schemes.
  - Ethics Committee letter of approval (and possibly a copy of the submission, composition of the Committee and its constitution).
  - The planned patient information leaflet and consent form if these differ from those suggested by the Sponsor.
  - Any necessary registration documents, e.g. to national or hospital authorities.
  - Financial agreement.
  - Signed letter of indemnity (where applicable).
- The following documentation should be received from an external Sponsor before the start of the study:
  - At least one copy of the Investigator's Brochure or equivalent (see SOP 8: Investigator's Brochure). In a Phase IV study the data sheet information may be provided instead.
  - At least one copy of the study protocol.
  - Examples of the patient information and consent forms.
  - An example of the CRF.
  - A contract detailing the terms and conditions for performing the trial, including the financial agreement.
  - Documentation of the insurance or indemnity arrangements for the study or letter of indemnity should be discussed and agreed.
- Recruitment rates should be discussed and agreed with the Monitor and a recruitment strategy decided upon (see SOP 14: Patient Recruitment and Intention to Enrol).
- Emergency contact telephone numbers should be obtained from the Monitor, particularly in double blind trials, so that contact is possible 24 hours a day, where required.

SOP approved by: _____

Signature: _____ *Date:* _____

SOP 13 – CHECKLIST 1
Pre-study Monitoring Visits

Protocol Code: [   ]   Date of Protocol: | | | | |
                                                     dd mm yy

Abbreviated Title: _____

Sponsor Name: _____

To be completed after each pre-study visit by the Monitor

Date of meeting: | | | | | | | | | Duration: | | | | | |
                  day   month year   hh   mm

	Yes	No	Comments (see end) (comment no.)
Is it the final version of the protocol?	☐	☐ *	☐

If no, draft number: [   ]

	Yes	No	Comments (see end) (comment no.)
Has the study protocol checklist been completed?	☐	☐	☐
Is the study protocol acceptable?	☐	☐	☐
Are the other terms and conditions acceptable?	☐	☐	☐
Are there any outstanding issues?	☐	☐	☐
Name of institute or department where the data will be analysed:			_____
What plans are there for publishing the results of the study?			_____

	Yes	No	Comments (see end) (comment no.)
Will the centre be involved in checking the draft CRFs?	☐	☐	☐
Are the compensation arrangements satisfactory?	☐	☐	☐
Is the financial agreement acceptable?	☐	☐	☐

Checklist completed by: _____ *on* _____

(date)

SOP 13 – CHECKLIST 1
Pre-study Monitoring Visits

Comments (Number the comments in the left-hand column)

SOP 13 – CHECKLIST 2
Pre-study Monitoring Visits

Protocol Code: [＿＿＿＿＿＿]   Date of Protocol: | | | | | |
                                                  dd mm yy

Abbreviated Title: _____

Sponsor Name: _____

To be completed after the study start meeting

Date of study start meeting: | | | | | | | | | Duration: | | | | | |
                               day   month   year   hh   mm

List here the names of all the staff who attended the meeting:

name	**name**
_____	_____
_____	_____
_____	_____
_____	_____
_____	_____

	Yes	No	Comments (see end) (comment no.)
Is there anyone on the study team checklist who did not attend the study start meeting?	☐ *	☐	☐

*If yes, the study responsible person must ensure that they are informed about the relevant aspects of the study.

Documentation given to Sponsor	Date given to Sponsor			Comments (see end) (comment no.)
Curriculum vitae of Principal Investigator				☐
	day	month	year	
Curriculum vitae of Sub-Investigator				☐
	day	month	year	
Ethics Committee approval				☐
	day	month	year	
Laboratory reference ranges, and QA/QC documentation				☐
	day	month	year	

SOP 13 – CHECKLIST 2
Pre-study Monitoring Visits

	Day	Month	Year	Comment
Ethics Committee composition	⊔⊔ day	⊔⊔ month	⊔⊔ year	☐
{Registration documents} enter N/A if not applicable	⊔⊔ day	⊔⊔ month	⊔⊔ year	☐
Financial agreement	⊔⊔ day	⊔⊔ month	⊔⊔ year	☐

Documentation from Sponsor	**Date received by Investigator**			**Comments** (see end) (comment no.)
Investigator's Brochure/data sheet information	⊔⊔ day	⊔⊔ month	⊔⊔ year	☐
Study protocol (final version)	⊔⊔ day	⊔⊔ month	⊔⊔ year	☐
Patient information and consent form	⊔⊔ day	⊔⊔ month	⊔⊔ year	☐
Example of the CRF	⊔⊔ day	⊔⊔ month	⊔⊔ year	☐
Contract/financial agreement/terms and conditions	⊔⊔ day	⊔⊔ month	⊔⊔ year	☐
Copy of the insurance policy for the study or other details of compensation	⊔⊔ day	⊔⊔ month	⊔⊔ year	☐

	Yes	**No**	**Comments** (see end) (comment no.)
Delivery of study medication and materials arranged?	☐	☐	☐
Have study drugs been delivered?	☐	☐	

If yes, where located? _____

If no, what are the proposed arrangements? _____

	Yes	**No**	
Have CRFs and other data collection material been delivered?	☐	☐	

If yes, where located? _____

If no, what are the proposed arrangements? _____

Checklist completed by: _____ *on* _____

(date)

SOP 13 – CHECKLIST 2
Pre-study Monitoring Visits

<u>Comments</u> (Number the comments in the left-hand column)

SOP 14
Patient Recruitment and Intention to Enrol

Background

Patient Recruitment

The first step is to define exactly what is meant by patient recruitment. This is not as straightforward as it sounds. There are several steps from the patient being identified and contacted to starting the study treatment. These include screening the patient, obtaining informed consent, randomising the patient, a possible baseline assessment and then initiation of treatment. Exactly when the patient is said to be enrolled in the trial should be defined in the protocol.

The recruitment period, i.e. starting and finishing date of recruitment for the entire study, may also be defined in the protocol.

Intention to Enrol list

For the purpose of this SOP, an 'Intention to Enrol list' is a record of all patients who were considered, were eligible for the study, but who, for one reason or another, were not included. This list enables a comparison of the potential patient population with the patient population actually enrolled in the study. It is helpful when questions of bias arise during evaluation of the data.

SOP 14
Patient Recruitment and Intention to Enrol

Purpose

To describe the procedure for recruiting patients into the study, and entry of patients in the Intention to Enrol list.

Other Related Procedures

SOP 9: Estimation of Patient Numbers
SOP 13: Pre-study Monitoring Visits
SOP 5: Review and Validation of the Protocol
SOP 15: Obtaining Personal Written Informed Consent
SOP 17: Randomisation and Stratification

Procedure

1. Who?

The Principal Investigator or study responsible person must discuss the recruitment strategy with the Monitor during the pre-study monitoring visits.

One of the Investigators, or the Study Site Co-ordinator if available, will be responsible for keeping records of patient recruitment and will inform the Principal Investigator and the Monitor of progress with recruitment.

The exact procedure for patient recruitment should be detailed in the study protocol; this must be checked by the Principal Investigator. All Investigators must be completely familiar with the recruitment procedure.

2. When?

Before the first patient is enrolled a recruitment strategy should be planned. Recruitment rates must be regularly assessed during the recruitment period, with reassessment of the strategy when targets are not being met.

The actual recruitment procedure should be performed every time a potential patient comes to the clinic.

3. How?

- According to the protocol and the preferences of the department, it must be decided whether all the patients will be recruited in one block, several blocks or sequentially.

SOP 14
Patient Recruitment and Intention to Enrol

- By estimation of likely patient numbers, and accounting for the length of the recruitment period, recruitment goals should be set. For example, if you have estimated that you can bring 20 patients into the study and the recruitment period is six months, you must enrol approximately four patients per month. You must make allowance for possible slower recruitment at the beginning of the study and also for holidays etc.
- Every patient who is considered a potential candidate for the study should be entered in an Intention to Enrol list. They should be entered on this list regardless of how likely you think they are to give their consent.
- The next step is to obtain the patient's informed consent according to SOP 15: Obtaining Personal Written Informed Consent. In some studies, the screening tests for the study will be done before informed consent is obtained. Reference must be made to the protocol for specific details. Normally the patient will then be randomised after consent has been obtained. Note that in double blind studies neither the patient nor the Investigator will know the treatment allocation at the time when the patient gives the informed consent.
- After randomisation enter the patient's code/ID number in the Intention to Enrol list. The Intention to Enrol list can then serve as the coded patient list, which must be archived at the end of the study. If there is no Intention to Enrol list planned in the study, a record must be kept of all patients randomised in the trial, with patient name, year of birth and treatment allocation or treatment package number.

SOP approved by: _____

Signature: _____ *Date:* _____

SOP 14 – CHECKLIST
Patient Recruitment and Intention to Enrol

Protocol Code: [_____]   Date of Protocol: |__|__|__|
                                                    dd mm yy

Abbreviated Title: _____

Sponsor Name: _____

How many patients do you plan to enrol in the study? [_____] *
*see checklist in SOP 9: Estimation of Patient Numbers

What is the planned method of recruitment?

Block recruitment ☐

Sequential recruitment ☐

If sequential recruitment:

How long is the recruitment period? [_____] days, weeks, months

What is the planned recruitment rate
for the department? [_____] patients per ___

	Yes	**No**	**Comments** (see end) (comment no.)
Is there a flowchart in the protocol detailing recruitment procedure?	☐	☐ *	☐

*If no, complete the flowchart provided

	Yes	**No**	**Comments** (see end) (comment no.)
Are there any foreseeable problems with the procedure?	☐	☐	☐
Does the Sponsor need to be notified of subjects entered at the time of enrollment?	☐	☐	

If yes, what is the procedure? _____

_____

Checklist completed by: _____ *on* _____
                                                    (date)

SOP 14 – CHECKLIST
Patient Recruitment and Intention to Enrol

Insert the appropriate terms from the following list in the diagram below:

Enter patient in Intention to Enrol list

Obtain informed consent

Perform screening tests for inclusion/exclusion criteria

Perform additional screening tests

Randomisation ($\pm$ Stratification)

Enter patient code in Intention to Enrol list, or reason why not included in the study

Baseline assessment

Start treatment

Flowchart completed by: _____ *on* _____

(*date*)

SOP 14 – CHECKLIST
Patient Recruitment and Intention to Enrol

Comments (Number the comments in the left-hand column)

SOP 15
Obtaining Personal Written Informed Consent

Background

Informed consent in the context of clinical trials may be regarded as: The voluntary confirmation of a subject's willingness to participate in a particular trial and the documentation thereof.

It is morally unacceptable to perform clinical research on someone without first informing them and obtaining their consent.

To quote the Declaration of Helsinki: 'In any research on human beings, each potential subject must be adequately informed of the aims, methods, anticipated benefits and potential hazards of the study and the discomfort it may entail. He or she should be informed that he or she is at liberty to abstain from participation in the study and that he or she is free to withdraw his or her consent to participation in the study at any time. The physician should then obtain the subject's freely given informed consent, preferably in writing.'

The EC Guidelines state that: 'The information to the patient should be given in oral and written form wherever possible' . . . and . . . 'subjects must be allowed sufficient time to decide whether or not they wish to participate.'

The ICH GCP Guideline naturally maintains these requirements, but also states that: 'the Investigator, or a person designated by the Investigator, should fully inform the subject' and that the written consent forms should be signed 'by the person who conducted the informed consent discussion'.

The words underlined are those often considered of particular importance when obtaining written informed consent.

Obtaining written informed consent can be a controversial issue for Study Site Co-ordinators (SSCs) who are not medically qualified. The Declaration of Helsinki clearly states that the person obtaining the informed consent should be a qualified physician. Many SSCs, however, do obtain written informed consent from study subjects. Suffice to say if you are obtaining written informed consent and are not medically qualified our advice is:

- Ensure that your Local Research Ethics Committee is aware that you are obtaining consent.
- If you are a nurse and/or a member of a professional organisation ensure that the organisation is aware, and if necessary has advised you.
- Be fully informed and familiar with the information you are giving to the study subject. This is particularly important for the patient information sheet, especially if it is written by the sponsoring company (see Points to note).

Points to note

It is very important that the Investigator/Sub-Investigator/SSC is fully familiar with the study protocol, patient information sheet and consent form before written informed consent is obtained. This is particularly important for new Research Registrars or SSCs newly employed to run a study.

SOP 15
Obtaining Personal Written Informed Consent

Informed written consent should not be obtained by a person who is not medically qualified or by a locum doctor. All persons who obtain written informed consent must have a copy of their CV in the Investigator file for the specific study which must be kept up to date.

The patient information sheet and consent form used to obtain written informed consent must be the same as the forms approved by the Local Research Ethics Committee. Any alterations subsequent to this approval to any of the forms must be submitted to the Ethics Committee and passed by them before they are used. To help ensure this, all patient information sheets and consent forms should be identified by the date of the version.

SOP 15
Obtaining Personal Written Informed Consent

Purpose

This SOP describes the procedure for obtaining personal written informed consent from a study subject. This involves ensuring that they understand what they are signing by means of a verbal explanation and a written patient information sheet. This SOP describes the two phases.

If the patient is unable to give personal written informed consent then SOP number 16 applies.

Other Related Procedures

SOP 16: Obtaining Informed Consent for Patients Unable to Give Personal Consent
SOP 5: Review and Validation of the Protocol

Procedure

1. Who?

- Verbal explanation of the study can be given by an SSC or a doctor.
- A medically qualified person is the only person who will obtain the written consent. This must be the Investigator or an approved member of the study team.

(A point to note here: Before the medically qualified person obtains the written informed consent they must be sure in their own mind that the person consenting to the study understands what it entails.)

2. When?

Written informed consent must be obtained before any study-specific procedures are undertaken.

3. How?

- Potential study subjects, i.e. those thought to fulfil the inclusion/exclusion criteria of the study, will be identified. The potential patient will initially be approached by either the physician or the SSC. They introduce themselves, saying for example, 'Hello, my name is . . . and I am a nurse/doctor/research assistant; could I come and have a chat with you?'
- A description of the study will be given to the patient verbally using non-technical language and if necessary using diagrams. It is helpful if the patient's relative or friend is present and they should be encouraged to join in the conversation. This initial contact is important and every attempt should be made by the physician/SSC to answer any questions the potential study subject and/or the relative or friend may ask.

SOP 15

Obtaining Personal Written Informed Consent

- When describing the study the physician/SSC should cover the following:
  - That it is a research procedure, and which aspects are experimental – it may or may not be beneficial to the subject – e.g. placebo.
  - The purpose of the trial.
  - Details about the drug under investigation. If there is a placebo arm to the study, this must be carefully explained.
  - The design of the trial, for example 'double dummy' or 'crossover'. Often a diagram is helpful here.
  - The number of people involved.
  - Duration of the trial. If the trial is a long-term one, enthusiasm is required.
  - Number of visits involved and duration of the visits. The area where the patient will be seen and by whom.
  - Procedures involved, for example blood tests, ECGs, urine samples and chest x-rays – how many and how often.
  - The responsibilities of the subject if he/she participates.
  - Out of pocket expenses and the receipt procedure. If a taxi account is set up for the study, then this will be explained. If payments are entailed, the details must be covered, including the arrangements for pro-rated payments.
  - The risks involved to the subject and any benefit that might be expected. If no clinical benefit is intended, the subject must be told.
  - Questions about the patient's medical history will be asked and disclosure of all medication the patient is taking, which will be kept up to date if changes occur.
  - Alternative procedures or treatments.
  - If the study has a specific exclusion criterion, for example a left ventricle ejection fraction <35%, but this is measured only after the patient has given written consent, this exclusion will be carefully explained. Providing written informed consent does not mean definite progression into the study.
  - The availability of compensation and treatment if needed.
  - That, because it is a study, written consent is needed which is voluntary and there is no penalty for refusal.
  - The right to withdraw from study medication at any time without affecting their future medical care. Similarly, if the Investigator thinks that the study medication is not suiting the patient, then the medication would be stopped.

Obtaining Personal Written Informed Consent

- If the patient is withdrawn from study medication for whatever reason that the site would still like to keep 'in touch' with the study patient – this could be via the telephone.
- Participation is confidential; the patient will usually be known only by initials and a special number. However, authorised representatives from regulatory bodies, the pharmaceutical company (Sponsor) and the Ethics Committee will have access to patients' records. If the study is within the UK and involves the Office of Population Census and Surveys this confidential procedure will be explained to the patient.
- 24-hour emergency number explained.
- At the end of the verbal explanation the subject will be asked for an initial reaction to what has been told to them. This usually comes in the form of three responses:
  - A definite no. The researcher says thank you for taking the time to listen and departs.
  - Unsure. The researcher will leave a patient information sheet with the potential study subject saying something like: 'What I have told you is written down on this information sheet. My name and the telephone number where you can contact me are written on the bottom of the page: do not hesitate to phone me if you have any further questions. I will call back to see you on . . .' Here the researcher will give a date and time convenient to the potential study subject. The researcher will say before they depart something like: 'Feel under no pressure to join the study, if you decide not to join then it will not affect your future care in any way.'
  - Yes. The researcher will give the patient a patient information sheet for the study on which will be written down all that the researcher has described to the patient. The researcher will then give the potential study subject the opportunity to read the information sheet. Depending on the type of study, the researcher may give the patient a clinic appointment to return in a week's time so that the potential study subject has ample time to consider the study. If the study is an acute study, then the researcher will ask the patient, after giving them the opportunity to read the patient information sheet, if they are still willing to participate in the study and to sign the consent form.
- After the potential study subject has had the study explained verbally and has had the opportunity to ask any questions and is satisfied that their questions have had a satisfactory answer, the physician will ask the subject to provide a signature on the consent form, which may be in triplicate: one copy for the patient to keep with the information sheet, one copy for the patient notes, the third copy to be kept in the study Investigator file. The best consent forms are often the ones that are attached to the patient information sheet. However this is sometimes not possible. The consent form will have the following information on it:
  - Study title and number.
  - A statement to say that the subject has had the study explained to them by . . . and had the potential risks benefits and alternative therapies, if any, explained to them.

SOP 15
Obtaining Personal Written Informed Consent

- The signature is voluntary, and they are free to withdraw at any time and need not have to give an explanation for withdrawal.
- That their medical records may be reviewed by authorised personnel. That confidentiality will be maintained at all times. Any written reports of the study will not mention them by name.
- Compensation guidelines and treatments should the study subject be injured or disabled whilst participating in the trial.
- The consent form should be signed and dated by the following people:
    - A medically qualified person providing the information, this being the Investigator or Sub-Investigator.
    - The subject.
    - A witness, if this is possible and if required for the study. A witness is defined as someone who records that the subject has provided consent of their own free will and has been fully informed of the study. The best witness is a subject's friend or family member who has sat in when the study was being explained to the patient. A witness must have no vested interest in the study; therefore a research assistant/ SSC/Sub-Investigator is not suitable as a witness.
- All signatures should be dated by the person who is signing and under the signature they should write their name in block capitals.

SOP approved by: _____

Signature: _____ *Date:* _____

SOP 15 – CHECKLIST 1
Obtaining Personal Written Informed Consent

Protocol Code: [   ]   Date of Protocol: ⌊_⌋_⌋_⌋
                                                   dd mm yy

Abbreviated Title: _____

Sponsor Name: _____

1. Persons responsible for obtaining consent who have read *and are familiar with and understand the study protocol* and the patient information sheet

Signature   Initials   Designation   ✓ if Copy of CV   Authorisation by
                                         in Investigator file   Principal Investigator

                                                              Version and Date
                                                                     Approved
2. Consent and patient information sheet approved by Ethics Committee
(Please staple information sheet and consent form to the back of this checklist) _____

3. Procedure check
    Identify study subject
    Introduction and verbal explanation of the study remembering to cover the following:
        research procedure, experimental aspects
        purpose of trial
        placebo if necessary and details of drug
        trial design (dummy/crossover)
        number of subjects
        duration
        number of visits
        procedures
        responsibilities
        expenses
        risks and benefits
        medical history
        alternatives
        any study-specific exclusions after consent
        compensation
        voluntary
        right to withdraw at any time but to keep in touch if randomised
        confidentiality issues
        contact phone number

4. Signatures required on the consent form
    Researcher (medically qualified) – sign and date
    The subject – sign and date
    Witness (if required/possible) – sign and date

SOP 15 – CHECKLIST 2
Obtaining Personal Written Informed Consent

Protocol Code: [_____]   Date of Protocol: [| | |]
                                                    dd mm yy

Abbreviated Title: _____

Sponsor Name: _____

The following checklist should be used if you are writing an informed consent form for your study and can also be used to check the content of an informed consent form drafted by the Sponsor.

Content of informed consent forms:	OK	Not OK	Comments (see end) (comment no.)
That this is research	☐	☐	☐
Details of experimental aspects	☐	☐	☐
The aim of the study	☐	☐	☐
Expected benefits for the patient and/or others	☐	☐	☐
Details of the comparative treatments and/or placebo	☐	☐	☐
Risks and inconveniences – e.g. invasive procedures, number of visits	☐	☐	☐
Responsibilities of the subject	☐	☐	☐
Explanation of any alternative/standard therapies	☐	☐	☐
Refusal to participate, or withdrawal at any stage, without subsequent disadvantages	☐	☐	☐
Scrutiny of personal information during audit and inspection	☐	☐	☐
Confidentiality of all personal information	☐	☐	☐
Information about the procedures for compensation and treatment in case of injury or disablement	☐	☐	☐
Contact phone number	☐	☐	☐

The following checklist should be completed before enrolment of the first patient for all studies:

SOP 15 – CHECKLIST 2
Obtaining Personal Written Informed Consent

	Yes	No	Comments (see end) (comment no.)
Has the information and consent form been examined and approved by the Ethics Committee?	☐	☐	☐
Will any patients be unable to give personal informed consent?	☐	☐	☐
If yes, has the procedure been approved by the Ethics Committee?	☐	☐	☐
Is the informed consent form in a language that the patients can understand?	☐	☐	☐
Protocol checked and/or flowchart available, detailing when informed consent to be obtained?	☐	☐	☐
Time and duration of informed consent to be completed on consent form?	☐	☐	☐
In long trials: Will consent be repeated at intervals during the trial?	☐	☐	☐
Will informed consent be obtained using a different procedure to that in the SOP?	☐	☐	☐

* If yes, what procedure will be used? (oral information, oral consent, signed by witness only, randomised consent etc.)

```
                                                                           



```

Checklist completed by: _____ *on* _____
(date)

Checklist 2: Review of Consent Forms 2/3   113

SOP 15 – CHECKLIST 2
Obtaining Personal Written Informed Consent

Comments (Number the comments in the left-hand column)

SOP 16
Obtaining Informed Consent for Patients Unable to Give Personal Consent

Background

From the Declaration of Helsinki:

'In case of legal incompetence, informed consent should be obtained from the legal guardian in accordance with the national legislation. Where physical or mental incapacity makes it impossible to obtain informed consent, or when the subject is a minor, permission from the responsible relative replaces that of the subject in accordance with the national legislation.

Whenever the minor child is in fact able to give a consent, the minor's consent must be obtained in addition to the consent of the minor's legal guardian.'

The ICH GCP Guidelines allow for the subject's involvement in trials when unable to provide informed consent when the consent is given by the 'subject's legally acceptable representative'.

The European GCP Guidelines state that when 'the subject is incapable of giving personal consent the inclusion of such patients may be acceptable if the Ethics Committee is, in principle, in agreement and if the Investigator is of the opinion that participation will promote the welfare and interest of the subject. The agreement of a legally valid representative that participation will promote the welfare and interest of the subject should also be recorded by a dated signature. If neither signed informed consent nor witnessed signed verbal consent are possible, this fact must be documented with reasons by the Investigator.'

In life threatening situations and where there is no other approved or generally recognised therapy, it may be desirable to use a study medication. There may not, however, be sufficient time to obtain consent from the patient's legally valid representative. If, in planning a clinical study, such a situation is anticipated, the Ethics Committee must first approve the procedure. If, for such reasons, informed consent is not obtained, you must document it, with reasons.

SOP 16

Obtaining Informed Consent for Patients Unable to Give Personal Consent

Purpose

This procedure should be used when a patient is incapable of giving informed consent. This may be, for example, because of unconsciousness or mental illness or disability such that the patient is unable to communicate or to understand enough to make an informed decision.

Other Related Procedures

SOP 5: Review and Validation of the Protocol
SOP 15: Obtaining Personal Written Informed Consent

Procedure

1. Who?

The Principal Investigator must ensure that the informed consent procedure is presented to the Ethics Committee and approved, e.g. who may act as a legally acceptable representative in the country where the study is to take place.

Otherwise, as for normal informed consent.

2. When?

As for normal informed consent.

3. How?

The same procedure for normal informed consent should be followed with the legally acceptable representative of the subject.

If it is an emergency situation and there is no time to obtain consent from a legally valid representative, then this must be documented, with reasons. Note that this is only possible when the participation in the study will promote the welfare and interest of the subject.

SOP approved by: _____

Signature: _____ *Date:* _____

SOP 16 – CHECKLIST
Obtaining Informed Consent for Patients Unable to Give Personal Consent

Protocol Code: [　　　　]   Date of Protocol: |　|　|　|
                                                  dd mm yy

Abbreviated Title: _____

Sponsor Name: _____

Yes/No

Does the protocol permit entry of patients unable to give
written informed consent themselves?   ☐

Are any details given in the protocol?   ☐

If yes, give details here: _____

Note name of any patient for whom consent was given by a legally acceptable representative	Reason not consented personally	Name of acceptable representative

Checklist completed by: _____ *on* _____
                                                          (date)

SOP 17
Randomisation and Stratification

Background

Most clinical trials are randomised trials. Randomisation is basically the haphazard (i.e. by equal chance) allocation of patients to one of two or more different treatment regimens. The reasons for randomisation are well described in Pocock's book, *Clinical Trials, A Practical Approach*, Chapter 4. It is well worth reading a little on the subject and understanding the principles behind randomisation – as an Investigator you should satisfy yourself that it is ethically and clinically acceptable to submit your patients to the randomisation procedure. If for any reason you are not happy with randomising patients according to a particular protocol, you should not act as Investigator in the study.

Stratification is a modification of the randomisation procedure, usually used in smaller trials, where the aim is to avoid differences between treatment groups which may occur by chance.

For example, it may be known that people over the age of 30 respond better to a particular treatment than people under 30. During the randomisation process, it may occur by chance that significantly more younger people are in one treatment group than the other, which could obviously affect the evaluation of the results.

Stratification is therefore a modification of the randomisation procedure which ensures that approximately equal numbers of in this case people over 30 and people under 30 are allocated to each treatment group. You should note that it is only meaningful to stratify according to factors which would affect the outcome of the trial, and not according to factors which are just clinically interesting, e.g. on tumour histology if this were thought to have no influence on outcome.

Randomisation and stratification procedures differ widely from study to study. They may involve phoning or faxing a central randomisation office, or may consist of a package of sealed envelopes provided by the Sponsor to each study site. Double blind studies may have quite elaborate procedures. Exact details will be included in the protocol and you should refer to the procedure there.

If the procedure is ambiguous or you are not familiar with it, ask the Monitor for clarification.

SOP 17
Randomisation and Stratification

Purpose

To describe the procedure during randomisation and stratification.

Other Related Procedures

SOP 5: Review and Validation of the Protocol
SOP 14: Patient Recruitment and Intention to Enrol

Procedure

1. Who?

The people involved in planning the study and writing the protocol will decide the methods, if any, to be used. The Principal Investigator may be involved at this stage.

All Investigators and other staff involved in patient recruitment must be familiar with the randomisation procedure for the particular study.

2. When?

Randomisation and stratification procedures should be defined as part of the protocol and agreed before the protocol is finalised.

3. How?

- The protocol must be reviewed at a pre-study meeting to assess the randomisation procedures.
- The attached checklist should be completed as documentation of the procedure.
- Ambiguities in the documentation of the procedure should be resolved with the Sponsor and the documentation clarified (for example by attaching a revised completed checklist).

SOP approved by: _____

Signature: _____ *Date:* _____

SOP 17 – CHECKLIST
Randomisation and Stratification

Protocol Code: [＿＿＿＿＿]　　　Date of Protocol: | | | |
　　　　　　　　　　　　　　　　　　　　　　　　　dd mm yy

Abbreviated Title: ＿＿＿＿＿＿＿＿＿＿＿＿＿＿＿＿＿＿＿＿＿

Sponsor Name: ＿＿＿＿＿＿＿＿＿＿＿＿＿＿＿＿＿＿＿＿＿

Yes/No

Is trial randomised?　　　☐

Is trial stratified?　　　☐

If yes, give details: ＿＿＿＿＿＿＿＿＿＿＿＿＿＿＿＿＿＿＿＿＿＿

＿＿＿＿＿＿＿＿＿＿＿＿＿＿＿＿＿＿＿＿＿＿＿＿＿＿＿＿＿＿＿

Describe randomisation procedure:

Does procedure involve telephoning a central number?　　　☐

　　Number: ＿＿＿＿＿＿　Contact name: ＿＿＿＿＿＿

　　or faxing a central number?　　　☐

　　Number: ＿＿＿＿＿＿　Contact name: ＿＿＿＿＿＿

Checklist completed by: ＿＿＿＿＿＿＿＿＿＿ *on* ＿＿＿＿＿＿＿＿＿
　　　　　　　　　　　　　　　　　　　　　　　　(date)

SOP 18
Blinding: Codes and Code Breaking

Background

Trials may be 'blinded' to avoid the introduction of bias. If patient, Investigator or statistician know which treatment the patient is receiving, it may influence response to the treatment, or the assessment of response and thus bias results. For example, if the Investigator gives a patient the new treatment, he/she may then observe the patient more closely or may communicate more positively with the patient. He/she may also evaluate the patient groups differently. If the patient knows they are receiving the new treatment and not the standard, this may also affect response (positively or negatively).

Placebos are often used when there is no standard therapy available, or the efficacy of the 'standard treatment' has not been established. When one group of patients receives treatment and the other receives nothing, it could be that the group on treatment shows an improvement compared to the control group. The problem is that you don't know if they showed the improvement just because they were being actively treated or whether it was due to a real effect of the substance, therapy or surgery. It has often been demonstrated that many minor illnesses could be effectively treated by placebos.

The reason for using placebo in clinical trials is therefore to attempt to make patient attitudes as similar as possible between the treatment groups. The patient should not be aware that they are receiving a placebo and therefore the trial should at least be designed as a trial that blinds the patient (single blind).

Double blind trials are those where neither the Investigator nor the patient know which treatment the patient is receiving. Most double blind trials involve therapy with a test treatment compared with a placebo. However, they can also consist of a test treatment and a standard treatment. To be properly blinded, the two blinded treatments must be perfectly matched for appearance, taste, smell etc. If this is not possible for practical reasons, a 'best attempt' is usually considered acceptable.

It is sometimes necessary to compare two treatments with different methods of application, e.g. comparing a tablet with a topical application. In this case it may be necessary to have a 'double dummy' design, i.e. one treatment group receives the test tablet with a placebo cream, the other group a placebo tablet with the test cream. Here each placebo must be matched with the respective test substance.

Blinding often complicates the randomisation procedure, and it is also necessary to have a coding procedure, identifying the patient number or the medication code number with the treatment. The patient number and medication code number may be the same.

In ophthalmological research the term *double masked* may be used, to avoid any disagreeable associations and possible confusion.

SOP 18
Blinding: Codes and Code Breaking

Purpose

To describe the procedure in blinded trials for dealing with the codes and when and how codes may be broken.

Other Related Procedures

SOP 17: Randomisation and Stratification
SOP 3: Study Files and Filing
SOP 20: Study Drugs

Procedure

1. Who?

The Sponsor of the clinical trial should plan and organise the procedures for blinding, randomisation, coding and possible code breaking. The details should be written in the study protocol (but obviously not in such detail that the code can be deciphered!).

The code should normally only be broken by the Principal Investigator after consultation with the Monitor/Sponsor. Where considered necessary, Sub-Investigators may also break the code.

2. When?

The code break procedure must be established before the first patient begins treatment.

The code should generally only be broken in the case of an adverse event where it is necessary for the Investigator to know which treatment the patient is receiving before the condition can be treated.

The code may also have to be broken if, for example, a child took the study medication.

Where possible, the Sponsor should be notified before the code is broken and in any case as soon as possible.

3. How?

- The exact procedure varies. The protocol must be reviewed and the procedure established. Normally the Principal Investigator must contact the Monitor or Sponsor before breaking the code. Whenever possible and certainly where required, ensure at the start of the study that 24-hour contact with the Sponsor is possible – obtain names and telephone numbers and keep them in an accessible place, known to all department staff.

SOP 18
Blinding: Codes and Code Breaking

- The codes may be contained in individual envelopes stored at the study site to be opened by the Investigator or the pharmacist, or the code may only be available via the Sponsor. All staff must know where any code envelopes are stored. Code envelopes will be checked by the Monitor during monitoring visits.
- When the code is broken for an individual patient, this must be documented on the CRF with the reasons for breaking the code. The code envelope that was opened should also be annotated with the reason.
- The Sponsor must be notified, by fax preferably or telephone and then in writing, as soon as possible.

SOP approved by: _____

Signature: _____ *Date:* _____

SOP 18 – CHECKLIST
Blinding: Codes and Code Breaking

Protocol Code: [_____]   Date of Protocol: |__|__|__|
dd mm yy

Abbreviated Title: _____

Sponsor Name: _____

Yes/No

Is trial blinded?   ☐

If yes, where are codes held? _____

Who has direct access to the codes? _____

How can they be contacted? _____

In the event of code break, who requires notification?

Name	Phone Number	Fax Number

Details of any codes broken during the course of the trial:

Subject Identifier(s)	Reasons for Code Break	Date Code Broken	Sponsor Contact Notified	
			Who?	When?

Checklist completed by: _____ *on* _____
(date)

SOP 19
Case Report Form (CRF) Completion

Background

In the European GCP Guidelines a CRF is defined as, 'a record of the data and other information on each subject in a trial as defined by the protocol'. The ICH GCP Guidelines say:

The reason for having CRFs in a study is to collect the necessary information about:

- the patients
- the administration of the study drug
- the outcome of the assessments.

CRFs are the official documentation of the trial for the authorities, and together with the source documents will be closely examined during audits and inspections.

The data on the CRFs will be entered into a computer system and the statistical analyses will then be performed.

The data on the CRFs is therefore the basis for the trial report and also for any publications, as well as making up part of the data for regulatory approval of a new drug.

SOP 19
Case Report Form (CRF) Completion

Purpose

To describe the procedure for completing, signing and correcting case report forms.

Other Related Procedures

SOP 2: Study Team: Definition of Responsibilities
SOP 3: Study Files and Filing
SOP 12: Laboratory

Procedure

1. Who?

Only the Investigator and Sub-Investigators including the Study Site Co-ordinator named in the Study File may complete CRFs. If stated in the Study File, laboratory, nursing and other personnel may complete specific pre-defined sections.

2. When?

CRFs should be completed as soon as possible after the patient assessment. Before any monitoring visits you should ensure that all CRFs are as up to date as possible.

3. How?

- When completing the form use a black ball point pen to complete the CRF. If the CRFs are printed on carbonless duplication paper, always make sure that a suitable separator is inserted under the form being completed.
- If for some reason you cannot complete part of the form, you shouldn't just leave a blank space – this is impossible for the people doing the data entry into the computer to interpret. Instead write *unknown, uncertain, missing* or *test not done* as appropriate, or similar unambiguous words. Avoid using the ambiguous phrase, 'not available'.
- The CRFs must be signed where indicated by the Principal Investigator to indicate that he/she believes they are complete and correct. Some Sponsors require a signature on each page of the CRF, some only a signature on the final page.

SOP 19

RF) Completion

is should be made as follows:
line – the incorrect entry should still be
ing fluid.

explanation of the correction if it is not

e used when it is necessary to make
n taken from the centre, and follow the

's reference range or some other range
gnificant variation from one assessment
l the significance noted on the CRF.
uld be entered without conversion from
y the units of measurement differ from

name should never appear on the CRF.
of patients in the study consisting of the
er (for more details see SOP 14: Patient
s must be archived by the Principal
SOP 26: Archiving).

SOP approved by: _____

Signature: _____ *Date:* _____

SOP 20
Study Drugs

Background

In the ICH GCP Guidelines, responsibility for accountability of investigational product at the site rests with the Investigator/Institution. However, the Investigator 'may assign some or all' of his or her duties 'to an appropriate pharmacist or another appropriate individual' under his or her supervision.

Records should be maintained 'of the product's delivery to the trial site, the inventory at the site, the use by each subject, and the return to the Sponsor or alternative disposition of unused products'.

As described in the first section of the book, large amounts of time and money are invested in drug development and there is naturally much competition between pharmaceutical companies. It is very important for the commercial interests of the company that details of an investigational drug and possible indications are kept confidential.

On a purely practical note, it is obviously important that everyone involved in the study knows where study drugs and supplies are kept. It is particularly important in double blind studies that the code is in some way accessible at all times. This is dealt with in a separate SOP (SOP 18: Blinding: Codes and Code Breaking).

Documentation of study medication is an important part of GCP, but it is often inadequately done. It is perhaps one of the most difficult areas for the Investigator to appreciate the reasons for the documentation – there are already so many forms to fill in and this may seem to be an unnecessary additional burden.

Study drugs are often not yet approved by the authorities, and their safety and efficacy are not fully researched – hence the clinical trial. It is important that you give the study medication only to patients or volunteers who have given their informed consent, and the only way this can be checked is with careful documentation of who received what, when, and that any discrepancies are accounted for.

Another important reason for exact documentation is that, in the event of doubts about the drug's safety or suitability of use and subsequent interruption of the trial, the Sponsor can locate and recover the entire batch of study drugs.

SOP 20
Study Drugs

Purpose

To describe the procedure for the receipt and storage of trial drugs at the study site, and the documentation of their location from the time of receipt to final removal (or destruction).

To describe the procedure for dealing with post-trial named-patient supply of trial medication.

Other Related Procedures

SOP 18: Blinding: Codes and Code Breaking

Procedure

1. Who?

The Investigator must assume ultimate responsibility for trial drugs, but should consider designating an adequately qualified individual, such as a pharmacist, the day to day responsibility.

The individual designated for the management of trial medication is responsible for ensuring adequate receipt, storage, dispensing of trial drugs and their final return to the external Sponsor or their destruction.

The Investigator and study responsible individual are responsible for ensuring adequate communication between any external Sponsor and the individual responsible for the management of trial medication.

The Investigator, or appropriate designee, is responsible for ensuring that subjects are allocated appropriate medication at the appropriate times in compliance with the protocol.

As appropriate, staff conducting follow-up visits are responsible for assessing subjects' compliance with trial medication (e.g. ensuring returned tablets are consistent with records on diary cards).

The study responsible individual, and the individual responsible for the management of trial medication, should ensure that drug accountability requirements are met to the satisfaction of any external Sponsor as required.

SOP 20
Study Drugs

2. When?

Proposed procedures for receipt, storage and dispensing of drugs should be discussed early on (at pre-study monitoring visits with the Monitor where there is an external Sponsor) and, if applicable, with individuals from the pharmacy department who will be involved with the trial. Agreement on procedures must be reached before delivery of the first batch of trial medication.

Documentation for tracking the disposition of drugs (drug accountability forms) should be agreed before entry of the first patient.

Drug accounting documentation should be completed on an ongoing basis: on arrival of supplies, each time drugs are dispensed, on return and when returned drugs are transported back to the supplier or are destroyed.

Agreement on the storing and transporting of surplus and returned medications and containers should be reached as soon as required by the party storing the returns (and the party storing the surplus if this is different).

Whether named-patient supply might be possible at the end of the study should be established before the first patient is asked to consent to take part in the trial. Potential requirement for named-patient supply should be established for each individual patient at the earliest opportunity prior to the patient's completion of the study medication. This is important to enable the provider of the drug to make the necessary arrangements.

3. How?

- The planned location of stored drugs must be established. This must be a secure area with restricted access, and conditions appropriate for the material on trial. The conditions of storage should be documented.
- The individual responsible for the receipt, storage and management of trial drugs must be agreed with the appropriate individual and the external Sponsor where there is one. Adequate communication between the relevant parties should be ensured.
- The individual responsible for management of trial medication should have easy access to relevant information about the trial and the drug (e.g. copies of the protocol and Investigator's Brochure).
- An approximate description of the trial medication should be elicited, including the way it is packed and how much space it will occupy. The labelling plans should also be discussed.

SOP 20
Study Drugs

- Arrangements for the receipt of medication at appropriate times and delivery points should be agreed between the responsible individual and the supplier (e.g. Sponsor).
- Receipt of each delivery of study medication must be documented at the study site and the supplier/Sponsor be notified in writing of receipt in accordance with their requirements.
- Procedures for requesting and accessing the study medication should be agreed; who will have direct access to the medication should be documented.
- Procedures for code break (unblinding of study medication) should be established for blinded trials and made known to staff involved in the trial.
- Methods and/or forms for documenting the movement of trial medication should be agreed with all involved parties: the individual responsible for management of trial medication, the Investigator or study responsible individual and the Sponsor where there is one. This should include the documentation of 'internal movement' (e.g. from Pharmacy to a location on a ward for immediate access), dispensing to subjects, receipt of returns from subjects. Details to be recorded should include the subject's identification, the date given to the subject, what was given, by whom; when returns were received back, what was returned, who checked it, explanation of any anomalies (such as drugs not taken, but not returned, breakages etc.). Batch (or serial) numbers should be noted, expiry dates and a record that subjects were given the doses specified in the protocol.
- Trial medication should be given to subjects only as specified in the protocol. If there are restrictions on who may give medication to subjects this should be documented. This may occur because of the nature of the drugs, local regulations or to help ensure blinding where this would otherwise be difficult.
- The individual giving the medication to the subject must ensure that the subject understands when and how to take the medication, and where necessary how to record the relevant details.
- If the protocol allows dosage adjustment or other flexibility of regime, the Investigator must determine, with the agreement of the external Sponsor where applicable, who may alter the subject's trial medication, and the named individuals should be documented.
- Procedures for checking subjects' compliance with trial medication should be agreed and documented (e.g. checking that diary card records are consistent with returns, measuring plasma or urine levels of drug). If required, an appropriate Standard Operating Procedure should be prepared. Problems with compliance should be documented, and if the protocol is not explicit about how to deal with subjects who do not comply with treatment, the Investigator (in conjunction with the external Sponsor where applicable) should determine whether the subject may stay in the trial or be withdrawn. The procedure for dealing with medication returned by subjects should be documented (e.g. Will it be returned directly to Pharmacy or to the Investigator or a Study Site Co-ordinator?; Will tablets be counted, inhalers be weighed etc.?; Where will it be stored or will it be destroyed?).

SOP 20
Study Drugs

- Where there is an external Sponsor, trial medication should be stored until arrangements are made with the Sponsor for collection or until agreement from the Sponsor that it can be destroyed. If it is to be destroyed without being returned to the Sponsor, destruction must be documented and documentation forwarded to the Sponsor.
- When all subjects have completed the trial medication and the records are complete, the individual responsible for management of the medication or the Investigator should ensure that the records are accurate and sign and date them as being so.
- Where there is an external Sponsor, the Monitor will require time and space to monitor the documentation and storage facility. The individual responsible for the management of trial drugs should be available to give time as reasonably required and ensure that space is available for the Monitor to work efficiently.
- Whether the study drug will be available on a named-patient basis should be established and if so, what the procedure is for requisitioning it.
- Whether there might be any interaction between the study drug and any post-trial treatment must be considered.
- The Investigator must establish who will be responsible for the post-trial care of the patient if it is not to be the Investigator him or herself.
- If any patient is to receive named-patient supply of the study drug, the procedure for monitoring the patient whilst on the treatment must be established and documented. This should include a frequency of follow-up acceptable to the Sponsor/supplier.

SOP approved by: _____

Signature: _____ *Date:* _____

SOP 20 – CHECKLIST 1
Study Drugs

Protocol Code: [   ]   Date of Protocol: | | | | |
dd mm yy

Abbreviated Title: _____

Sponsor Name: _____

Management of Study Drugs

Responsibility and Storage

Who will be responsible for study drugs? _____

What storage conditions are required? _____
(i.e. temperature, lighting etc.)

Planned date of delivery of first batch of study drugs: __ / __ / __

Where will study drugs be delivered? _____

Who is responsible for acknowledging receipt? _____

Where will study drugs be stored (record all locations
and indicate reasons for multiple storage)? _____
(NB These must be secure facilities)

Who will have direct access to study medication? _____

_____

What may returns consist of? _____

Who will receive returns from the subject? _____

Where will returned medication be stored? _____

What happens to returns (describe)? _____

_____

_____

(Include any tablet counts, weighing etc.)

What finally happens to returns/surplus medication?   Returned to supplier [ ]

Destroyed [ ]

Other (details) [ ]

_____

_____

SOP 20 – CHECKLIST 1
Study Drugs

External Sponsor

Is there an external Sponsor for this study?   Yes/No

If yes, Monitor must be informed of individual responsible for management of study medication.

☐ (when done)

Monitor should be satisfied with planned storage facility   ☐ (when agreed)

Pre-trial meeting or discussion arranged between Monitor and individual responsible for study medication.

Date __/__/__

Where will the Monitor be able to work to review drugs and drug accountability etc.?

Drug and Trial Information

Ensure individual responsible for study medication is provided with a protocol.

Date provided __/__/__

How will individual have access to information about the drug?
(e.g. own copy of Investigator's Brochure, own copy of
other documentation, access to Investigator's copy etc.)

Date provided __/__/__

Description of the trial medication and packaging arrangements
(i.e. presentation, number of items per dispensing,
number of dispensing packs etc.)

SOP 20 – CHECKLIST 1
Study Drugs

Description of labels: _____
(or stick sample label here)

Details of any problems identified with labels: _____

_____

Dispensing

Will study drugs be transferred from the main storage area
for any reason other than when dispensed to trial subjects?   Yes/No

If yes, give reason: _____

and location: _____

How will the transfer be documented? _____
(attach copy of any standard form prepared)

Describe procedure for requisition of study medication: _____

_____

_____

Will prescriptions be used?   Yes/No

If yes, attach copies   ☐ (when attached)

Have drug accountability forms been prepared that include
the minimum information required by the SOP?   Yes/No

If yes, attach copies   ☐ (when attached)

If no, give reasons: _____

Number of dispensings per patient required by protocol: _____

Any restrictions on who may give medication to subjects?   Yes/No

If yes, give details: _____

Is adjustment of the dosage of the trial medication permitted
as part of the protocol?   Yes/No

If yes, who is authorised to do this? _____

SOP 20 – CHECKLIST 1
Study Drugs

Compliance

What checks are there on subject compliance to medication?

( ) Tablet counts
( ) Diary card records
( ) Blood samples
( ) Urine samples
( ) Observed when taking
( ) Other (give detail)

Is a specific SOP required?   Yes/No

If yes, who will prepare it?   _____

Checklist completed by: _____ *on* _____
                                                              (date)

SOP 20 – CHECKLIST 2
Study Drugs

Protocol Code: [_____]   Date of Protocol: |__|__|__|
                                                  dd mm yy

Abbreviated Title: _____

Sponsor Name: _____

Who will be responsible for patients' post-trial care? _____

What plans are there for patients' post-trial medication? _____

_____

Will the study drug be available at the end of the trial?   ( ) No
                                                              ( ) Yes, Named-patient
                                                              ( ) Yes, Other (details)

_____

What is the procedure for arranging named-patient supply? _____

_____

_____

How will patients on named-patient supply be monitored? _____

_____

(Include details of how frequently they will be followed up)

List of patients on named-patient supply:

Name	Trial Number	Date Started

Checklist completed by: _____   Date: _____

                           _____   Date: _____

                           _____   Date: _____

SOP 21
Monitoring Visits

Background

For every study performed to GCP standards, it is a requirement that a Monitor visits you, to ensure that the trial 'is conducted, recorded, and reported in accordance with the protocol, Standard Operating Procedures (SOPs), Good Clinical Practice (GCP) and the applicable regulatory requirements.' In particular, that 'the rights and well-being of human subjects are protected' (ICH GCP Guidelines).

An important part of a monitoring visit is comparing the entries in the case report forms with the original source documents (e.g. laboratory results, patient record card, ECG print outs). This procedure is known as Source Document Verification (SDV). The exact procedure will vary from Monitor to Monitor and also from country to country. In certain countries, for example, Monitors are generally not allowed direct access to patient files. In other countries, the Monitor may only look at patient files if the patient has directly given his/her consent. It may be necessary to perform SDV using the 'back-to-back' method, i.e. the Monitor has the CRFs, the Investigator the source documents and the Monitor asks the Investigator about the facts written in the CRFs, for example, the Monitor will ask for the year of birth and will then check the Investigator's answer with the entry in the CRF.

The ICH GCP Guidelines encourage the use of 'direct access' by Monitors to perform SDV and state that written information provided to subjects should include explanation that the Monitor will be 'granted direct access to the subject's original medical records for verification of clinical trial procedures and/or data, without violating the confidentiality of the subject, to the extent permitted by the applicable laws and regulations.'

SOP 21
Monitoring Visits

Purpose

This procedure describes the preparation for and the procedure to follow during monitoring visits.

Other Related Procedures

SOP 19: Case Report Form (CRF) Completion

Procedure

1. Who?

Normally, monitoring visits will be arranged in advance by the Monitor with the Principal Investigator and/or other staff as appropriate, soon after the first patient is enrolled.

2. When?

Depending on the study, visits will probably take place approximately every four to six weeks during the study. Depending on the length of the study and its progress, this interval may be prolonged or shortened.

All relevant documents should generally be gathered together before the planned visit.

3. How?

- Preparation:
  - Where possible, all case report forms should be made up to date, including any outstanding corrections from the last visit.
  - Where possible, all source documents should also be available, including those from other departments, e.g. radiology, which may be relevant to the study.
  - A room or quiet desk should be set aside for the use of the Monitor during the visit.
  - Prepare details of numbers of patients screened and enrolled in the study and of any other outstanding business requiring discussion.
- During the visit:
  - Where required by the Monitor, the Principal Investigator should be available on the day of the visit and if possible the Co-Investigators. Of course if there is a Study Site Co-ordinator, he or she should also be available.
  - It is preferable that the Principal Investigator always be available for at least a proportion of each monitoring visit in most studies.

SOP 21
Monitoring Visits

- The Monitor will normally require time to go through the CRFs and associated source documents alone, with a meeting with the appropriate site staff afterwards to discuss any problems or outstanding business. Appropriate staff will make themselves available for such discussion.
- The Monitor may also wish to examine facilities at the study site and check storage of the study medication and drug accountability. If so, appropriate arrangements should be made in advance and the Monitor should be accompanied on visits to other departments as determined by the Monitor.
- If the visit is because of a severe or serious adverse event, or some other specific problem, the Monitor should inform you of any special requirements beforehand.
- After the visit:
  - Source documents should be returned to the respective departments.
  - Missing data should be obtained and corrections done promptly – they are easier to do when the points are fresh in your mind – don't leave it until the day before the next visit!

SOP approved by: _____

Signature: _____ *Date:* _____

SOP 21 – CHECKLIST
Monitoring Visits

Protocol Code: [_____]   Date of Protocol: [| | |]
                                                  dd mm yy

Abbreviated Title: _____

Sponsor Name: _____

The following points should be used to prepare for monitoring visits:

Date of next monitoring visit [| |]   [| |]   [| |]
                                day   month   year

Total number of patients in the study (now) [_____]

Number of new patients recruited since last visit [_____]

Number of new patients anticipated in next month [_____]

	Yes	No	Comments (see end) (comment no.)
Any outstanding business to discuss?	☐	☐	☐
Any adverse events/protocol violations?	☐	☐	☐
Are all CRFs up to date?	☐	☐	☐
Have all corrections been made since the last visit?	☐	☐	☐
Are all source documents available?	☐	☐	☐
Is the room/area available at the arranged time of the visit?	☐ *	☐	☐

*Room number/name: _____

	initials	initials	initials
Who will be available during the monitoring visit?	[		]	[		]	[		]

Post Visit

Names of Monitor and any accompanying colleagues _____
_____

Duration of visit _____ hours

	Yes	No	Details on next page
Any outstanding tasks as result of visit?	☐	☐	

Checklist completed by: _____ *on* _____
                                                      (date)

Checklist 1/2   141

SOP 21 – CHECKLIST
Monitoring Visits

Comments (Number the comments in the left-hand column)

SOP 22

Adverse Event and Serious Adverse Event Reporting

Background

With the introduction of the ICH GCP Guidelines there have been slight changes to the definitions of an adverse event and a serious adverse event as compared with what you were used to in the European GCP Guidelines, but in practice you are unlikely to notice.

The definition of an adverse event is: 'Any untoward medical occurrence in a patient or clinical investigation subject administered a pharmaceutical product and which does not necessarily have a causal relationship with this treatment.' This includes 'any unfavourable and unintended sign (including an abnormal laboratory finding), symptom or disease temporally associated with the study drug'. This may include, for example, a cold, or an accident.

The definition of a serious adverse event is one that is
> Fatal
> Life threatening
> Results in hospitalisation or prolongs hospitalisation
> Significantly disabling/incapacitating
> or
> Is a congenital anomaly/birth defect
> The European GCP Guidelines also include cancer and the FDA GCP Guidelines include overdose

All adverse events, both serious and non-serious, must be recorded by the researcher in the workbook or case record forms. A non-serious adverse event may develop into a serious adverse event so it is important that the Investigator is aware of the definitions of a serious adverse event.

The ICH GCP Guidelines state that: 'All serious adverse events should be reported immediately to the sponsor,' and that 'immediate reports should be followed promptly by detailed written reports.' The Investigator 'should also comply with the applicable regulatory requirement(s) related to the reporting of unexpected serious adverse drug reactions to the regulatory authority(ies) and the IRB/IEC' (Independent Ethics Committee). For the Sponsor's responsibilities regarding adverse event reporting, the ICH GCP Guidelines state that: 'The Sponsor should expedite the reporting to all concerned Investigator(s)/Institution(s), to the IRB(s)/IEC(s), where required, and to the regulatory authority(ies) of all adverse drug reactions (ADRs) that are both serious and unexpected.' You should consider it your duty to report all serious adverse *events* to the Sponsor and in general let the Sponsor determine whether the 'event' is a 'reaction', i.e. break the treatment code, and 'unexpected', i.e. not declared in the information about the drug.

An 'adverse' event is perhaps not the best terminology to use, the word 'event' may be a better word to use. Many people misunderstand the words 'adverse event', interpreting it as some disease that they personally class as an adverse event. To clarify the point, perhaps the best way to illustrate it is by an imaginary case study.

SOP 22
Adverse Event and Serious Adverse Event Reporting

Case Study

A hanging flower basket fell on a study subject's head whilst they were walking in town one day during the summer, resulting in the study subject falling down and becoming unconscious. The subject's partner called for an emergency ambulance. On arrival at a local hospital's Accident and Emergency Department, in which the patient regained consciousness but could not recall the event, an x-ray revealed a fractured skull. The subject's consciousness level at this point was deteriorating and after further tests a sub-dural haematoma was diagnosed, which was evacuated under general anaesthesia. Post-operative recovery was uneventful and progressing well until day four, when the patient developed acute dyspnoea at rest during visiting time. An emergency lung scan was arranged that confirmed a diagnosis of pulmonary embolism. The study subject was anticoagulated and was eventually discharged from hospital.

The reader may think that a hanging basket falling on a patient's head is not at all related to the study medication, although agreeing that the events that followed are to be classed as a serious adverse event. This is because the patient was hospitalised and hospitalisation was prolonged due to a pulmonary embolus.

When more information was obtained on the events which led to the hanging basket falling, relatives had noticed that the study subject's *normal* pattern of behaviour during the summer changed dramatically. After commencing study medication, relatives had noticed an increase in restlessness and wandering. Trips into town, which normally the patient did approximately twice a year, had become a daily event.

It is not the Investigator's job to draw conclusions, it is the Investigator's responsibility to report the event accurately and with sufficient detail for others to draw conclusions once all the evidence has been gathered. A postscript to this true story is that it was found that all the patients randomised to the active drug at the end of the study were found to have developed irritability.

SOP 22
Adverse Event and Serious Adverse Event Reporting

Purpose

To describe the procedure for eliciting and recording and reporting adverse events and serious adverse events.

Other Related Procedures

None

Procedure

1. Who?

All staff in contact with subjects are responsible for noting adverse events that are reported by the subject and making them known to appropriate staff (for example medical or nursing staff). Appropriate staff members should conduct study visits, or assessments, and ensure that all adverse events are elicited as far as possible.

The Principal Investigator should sign a written report of each serious adverse event forwarded to the Sponsor.

2. When?

At each visit, or study assessment, adverse events that might have occurred since the previous visit or assessment should be elicited.

Adverse events ongoing on completion of the study should be followed up as required by the protocol and as clinically indicated.

3. How?

Adverse Event

- Document event in an unambiguous way as far as possible. For example, the patient may say that they 'felt sick'. This can be interpreted in many ways: either they felt nauseated or they may have felt unwell, or they may even have been vomiting!
- Ask patient the date and start and stop time of event. If the patient cannot remember, then as near as possible – document in hospital notes for SDV.
- Document severity – this may be clarified by the Sponsor in the protocol.
- Action taken regarding study drug – if any.
- Document any treatment/medication given for the event.
- Document event outcome.

SOP 22
Adverse Event and Serious Adverse Event Reporting

- Events ongoing at study completion should be followed up as detailed in the protocol and as clinically indicated. As a minimum each subject with such an event should be contacted after the trial at least once.

Serious Adverse Events

1. All events will be documented as above. However, if they come under the following definitions then the event will be classed as a serious adverse event:

   > Fatal
   > Life threatening
   > Significantly disabling/incapacitating
   > Results in hospitalisation or prolongs hospitalisation
   > Congenital anomaly

2. Inform the Sponsor within 24 hours of the Investigator's knowledge of the event. How the information is forwarded to the Sponsor varies, but it will be fully explained in the study protocol, and these procedures must be followed.

3. Respond promptly to requests for follow-up information from the Sponsor or other actions such as notification of the Ethics Committee.

SOP 23
Nursing Procedures

Background

Every department conducting clinical trials employs standard procedures for dealing with subjects, samples, reports, equipment etc.

Not all of these will require documenting as a written Standard Operating Procedure. However, it is worth considering preparing a formal document for those procedures that would have to be taught to new members of the department.

SOP 23
Nursing Procedures

Purpose

The procedures below are examples to aid you in writing your own study-specific procedures.

Other Related Procedures

SOP 0: Preparation, Approval and Review of SOPs
SOP 24: Clinical Procedures

SOP for Application of Nitro-glycerine Ointment

Background

Topical nitro-glycerine is absorbed from the skin and has a systemic effect on the blood vessels causing vasodilatation and improving cardiac perfusion.

Who? and **When?** would be completed as appropriate for your department.

How?

- Take the patient's baseline blood pressure to compare it with later readings.
- Topical nitro-glycerine is prescribed in the UK by the inch and comes with a rectangular piece of ruled paper to be used in applying the medication. Squeeze the prescribed amount of ointment onto the ruled paper. Put on gloves if you wish to avoid contact with the medication.
- After measuring the correct amount of ointment, tape the paper, drug side down, directly to the skin. For increased absorption, the doctor may request that you cover the site with plastic wrap or a transparent semi-permeable dressing.
- After five minutes, record the patient's blood pressure. If it has dropped significantly and he/she has a headache, notify the doctor immediately. The doctor may reduce the dose. If the patient's blood pressure has dropped but they have no adverse reactions, instruct them to lie still until it returns to normal.

SOP for Reconstitution and Withdrawal of Medications from a Vial

Equipment needed: medication vial, vial or ampoule of an appropriate diluent, an iodophor or ethyl alcohol swab, a syringe, two needles of appropriate size and a filter needle, if available, to screen particulate matter that may accumulate from reconstitution.

Nursing Procedures

How?

- Place the medication vial on a level surface. Wipe the rubber diaphragm on the neck of the vial with the swab. Do not rub the diaphragm vigorously, because doing so can introduce bacteria from the non-sterile rim of the vial. Repeat the process with the vial of diluent.
- Next, pick up the syringe, uncap the needle, and pull back on the plunger until the space inside the syringe equals the amount of diluent desired. Puncture the rubber diaphragm of the diluent vial with the needle, and inject the air. Injecting the air creates a positive pressure within the vial and makes withdrawal of fluid easier as well as preventing a vacuum from forming after the contents are withdrawn.
- Invert the vial, and withdraw the desired amount of diluent. Next, inject the diluent into the medication vial and withdraw the needle. Roll or shake the vial to mix the medication thoroughly.
- If a filter needle is available, remove the first needle, attach the filter needle to the syringe and uncap it.
- If a filter needle is not available, leave the first needle attached to the syringe. Pull back the plunger until the volume of air in the syringe equals the volume of medication to be given.
- Puncture the diaphragm of the medication vial, and inject the air. Invert the vial, and withdraw the correct amount of solution. Replace the original needle or the filter needle with a clean sterile needle because medication that may have adhered to the needle when the solution was withdrawn from the vial can irritate the patient's tissues. The syringe filled with medication is now ready to label and administer to the patient.

SOP approved by: _____

Signature: _____ *Date:* _____

SOP 24
Clinical Procedures

Background

Every department conducting clinical trials employs standard procedures for dealing with subjects, samples, reports, equipment etc.

Not all of these will require documenting as a written Standard Operating Procedure. However, it is worth considering preparing a formal document for those procedures that would have to be taught to new members of the department.

SOP 24
Clinical Procedures

Purpose

The procedure below is an **example** procedure to aid you in writing your own study-specific procedures.

Other Related Procedures

SOP 0: Preparation, Approval and Review of SOPs
SOP 23: Nursing Procedures

SOP for Standardised Measurement of Blood Pressure

Procedure

1. Who?

The following staff (or grades of staff) are permitted to carry out this procedure: medically qualified staff, staff with nursing qualifications, trained technicians.

2. When?

The procedure should be carried out in accordance with times defined in the study protocol.

3. How?

To measure the blood pressure of a sitting patient, the patient must have been sitting down for the last five minutes. To measure the blood pressure of a standing patient, the patient must have been standing for the last two minutes.

The systolic blood pressure should be calculated from the mean of three consecutive measurements taken at one-minute intervals. None of the three measurements should deviate by more than 5 mmHg from the mean value.

- The blood pressure measurement should take place in a quiet room; the patient's arm should be held at heart level.
- The manometer should be at eye level so that the calibrations on the scale are easy to read.
- The cuff must be of adequate size. The width of the inflatable part should be at least 40%, the length at least 80% of the arm circumference.

SOP 24
Clinical Procedures

- Localise the brachial artery (medial upper arm) by palpation.
- Wrap the cuff carefully around the upper arm. The middle of the inflatable part should lie directly over the brachial artery. Do not rely on any markings on the cuff – check the midline yourself by folding the cuff in half. The lower edge of the cuff should be approximately 2.5 cm above the elbow.
- Ascertain the maximum inflation pressure by finding out the pressure with which the radial pulse is no longer palpable during rapid inflation of the cuff (palpable systolic pressure). The maximum cuff pressure is 30 mmHg above this value.
- Quickly and uniformly release the pressure. Wait 15 to 30 seconds before reinflating the cuff.
- Place the stethoscope over the elbow, underneath the cuff on the palpable brachial artery. The ear pieces of the stethoscope should be pointing forwards.
- The bell of the stethoscope should be applied with light pressure to ensure that the entire bell is in contact with the skin. Undue pressure can cause distortion of sounds.
- Inflate the cuff evenly and quickly to the maximum cuff pressure, as determined above.
- Release the cuff pressure at a rate of 2 to 3 mmHg per second.
- Read off the systolic blood pressure at the point where you hear at least two consecutive beats (Phase 1 of the *Korotkow* sounds).
- The blood pressure must always be given as an even number – read off at the next 2 mmHg marking.
- When the Phase V *Korotkow* sound is no longer audible, you can read off the diastolic blood pressure. Wait until the pressure is 10 to 20 mmHg lower to ensure that this sound is no longer audible and then quickly release the pressure.
- Make a note of the position of the patient (sitting or standing) and also of which arm was used to measure the blood pressure.
- Wait one minute and repeat the above procedure on the same arm. It is important to wait one minute to ensure that there is no remaining venous congestion.

SOP 24
Clinical Procedures

Specific problems:

Auscultatory gap

In some patients – especially those with hypertension – the normal sounds at high cuff pressure over the brachial artery can become temporarily silent during reduction of the pressure, only to reappear at lower cuff pressures. This early and temporary loss of pulse sounds is known as the auscultatory gap and occurs in the late stages of Phases I and II. This auscultatory gap can in certain circumstances be up to 40 mmHg, and there is therefore the danger of significantly underestimating the systolic pressure or overestimating the diastolic pressure. The existence of an auscultatory gap can be excluded by palpating the disappearance of the radial pulse during inflation of the cuff.

Effect of arm position

The blood pressure in the arm increases with the lowering of the arm below heart level, and decreases when the arm is raised. With indirect blood pressure measurement, the arm should be held so that the bell of the stethoscope is at heart level. Heart level is the mid point between the fourth intercostal space and left lower edge of the sternum. You should pay particular attention in standing patients to the position of the brachial artery in relation to the heart level. If the patient is lying on their back on a flat surface with a slightly raised head, it can be assumed that the brachial artery is at heart level. In sitting position, the arm should be placed on a table at a level just above the hips.

Patients with above average upper arm circumference (>41 cm)

When a standard cuff is used in patients with above average upper arm circumference, it can result in falsely elevated blood pressure measurements. This applies particularly when small cuffs are used, because the compressible soft tissue of the upper arm causes an excessive loss in cuff pressure. This problem can be minimised by the use of cuffs with a width of 40 to 50% of the measured upper arm circumference (or by excluding these patients from the study).

In patients who are not overweight, a normal adult cuff (width 15 cm) is adequate.

A blood pressure measurement on the lower arm is not recommended because falsely elevated blood pressure values often result.

SOP approved by: _____

Signature: _____ *Date:* _____

SOP 25
Trial Report

Background

At the end of the study, the data will be collected by the Sponsor (unless other arrangements have been made) and analysed by a biostatistician. A trial report should be written whether or not the trial has been completed. The report should include the following points:

- Identification of the study, including the allocated protocol number
- Name(s) of Investigator(s) and study site(s)
- When the study was conducted
- Objectives of the study
- Study design
- Description of the study population, including number of subjects studied
- Medication studied (or combination), including route of administration, dose, regimen and duration of treatment
- Results of study
- Study conclusions

For long term trials an annual report may be required by the authorities.

SOP 25
Trial Report

Purpose

To describe the procedure for agreeing the reporting of trial findings.

Other Related Procedures

SOP 26: Archiving

Procedure

1. Who?

The Principal Investigator and co-workers may be asked to check and/or sign the trial report.

2. When?

On completion of the final report.

You may be asked to assist in the writing of the final report. The division of responsibilities must be decided on before the start of the study, or as soon as possible.

3. How?

- The Principal Investigator together with the Co-Investigators must examine the report and check that it is an accurate record of the study. The Principal Investigator can then sign the report.
- The following points should be checked for accuracy before signing:
  - The description and numbers of the patient population are in accordance with the records at the department.
  - The methods described in the report reflect how the study was performed, including protocol violations and drop outs.
  - The incidence and nature of adverse events are accurately described.
  - The data have been analysed according to the methods described in the protocol, with all patients accounted for – including drop outs and protocol violations.
  - The conclusions drawn by the report, based on the results and the statistical analysis, are fair.

SOP 25
Trial Report

- It is obviously more difficult to assess the accuracy of the report in a multi-centre study, but it should reflect the experiences of your department.
- If there are any queries or inaccuracies in the report, resolve these with the Sponsor before signing.

SOP approved by: _____

Signature: _____ *Date:* _____

SOP 25 – CHECKLIST
Trial Report

Protocol Code: [   ]   Date of Protocol: | | | | |
                                                 dd mm yy

Abbreviated Title: _____

Sponsor Name: _____

It may be difficult to assess the accuracy of the report in a multi-centre study, but it should reflect the experiences of your department.

	Yes	No	Comments (see end) (comment no.)
Are the description and numbers of the patient population in accordance with the records at the department?	☐	☐	☐
Do the methods described reflect how the study was performed, including protocol violations and drop outs?	☐	☐	☐
Are the incidence and nature of adverse events accurately described?	☐	☐	☐
Have the data been analysed according to the methods described in the protocol, with all patients accounted for – including drop outs and protocol violations?	☐	☐	☐
Do you agree with the conclusions drawn by the report, based on the results and the statistical analysis?	☐	☐	☐
Are there any inaccuracies in the report?	☐ *	☐	☐
Are there any points which you feel require clarification?	☐ *	☐	☐

* If yes, give details on next page and discuss with Sponsor before signing:

Date of approval
of trial report: | | | | | | | | |
                   day   month   year   Signed by: _____

	Yes	No	Comments (see end) (comment no.)
Is it necessary to archive the trial report?	☐	☐	☐

Checklist completed by: _____ *on* _____
                                                              (date)

Checklist 1/2

SOP 25 – CHECKLIST
Trial Report

Comments (Number the comments in the left-hand column)

SOP 26
Archiving

Background

To ensure that results from clinical trials can be examined and checked at a later date it is necessary that both the Sponsor and the Investigator keep records of the trial. This can be important, for example, when unexpected side effects occur after the drug has been approved. The clinical trial data and source documents can be checked to examine any similar events that might have occurred during the trial.

The ICH GCP Guidelines have affected what must be archived at the study site and the period for which documents need to be retained. Prior to ICH GCP, many Sponsors routinely requested Investigators to retain all trial-related documents for 15 years after the completion of the trial. The European GCP Guidelines did not require this; merely that the patient codes (and patient names) be retained for 15 years and the remainder of the records for as long as the institution allows (in its usual practice).

The ICH GCP Guidelines are specific about which documents are essential for the conduct of a clinical trial, and which of these must be located in the Investigator's trial file. The ICH GCP Guidelines state that essential documents be retained 'until at least 2 years after the last approval of a marketing application in an ICH region', with a couple of additional caveats. This is not expected to be the sole responsibility of the Investigator; 'it is the responsibility of the Sponsor to inform the Investigator/Institution as to when these documents no longer need to be retained.'

SOP 26

Archiving

Purpose

To describe the procedure for archiving the study documents at the end of a clinical trial.

Other Related Procedures

SOP 3: Study Files and Filing

Procedure

1. Who?

The Principal Investigator must agree with the Sponsor the exact requirements for archiving and make or assist in making the necessary arrangements. If the Principal Investigator leaves the department during the archival period, he/she must make arrangements to transfer the responsibility to his/her successor and must also inform the Sponsor of the new arrangements.

2. When?

Although archiving occurs at the end of the study, the earlier the procedure can be agreed the better.

3. How?

- The coded patient list (patient full names together with year of birth and patient code number) must be archived, together with the patient consent forms, for as long as possible and for at least 15 years after completion of the trial.
- Essential documents as defined in the ICH GCP Guidelines will be retained until notification from the Sponsor is received that they no longer need to be retained.
- All data and documents should be made available if requested by relevant authorities.
- The patient source documents should be clearly marked that the patient has taken part in a clinical trial and that they should not be destroyed. After being so labelled they can then be archived in the hospital/clinic filing system.
- It may be arranged that the documentation be archived by the Sponsor. The details should be agreed with the Sponsor of the individual study. Access to the material should be restricted to the Investigator and the regulatory authorities.

SOP approved by: _____

Signature: _____ *Date:* _____

SOP 26 – CHECKLIST
Archiving

Protocol Code: [_____]   Date of Protocol: | | | |
                                                dd mm yy

Abbreviated Title: _____

Sponsor Name: _____

Date of study discontinuation/study end | | | | | | | | |
                                            day   month   year

Which of the following study site documents are to be archived at the study site?
(✓=Yes, X=No, NA=Does not apply)

Investigator's Brochure ☐ Amendments   ☐ Regulatory Approvals (e.g. CTX)   ☐
Signed Protocol ☐ Amendments   ☐ Principal Investigator's CV   ☐
Sample CRF (including revisions)   ☐ Sub-Investigator's CV   ☐
Sample Diary Card   ☐ Lab Reference Ranges   ☐
Sample Questionnaire   ☐ Lab Reference Ranges Updates   ☐
Consent Forms   ☐ Lab Quality Control Documentation (may not
Written Information for Subjects   ☐ be required)   ☐
Recruitment Advertisement   ☐ Instructions for Handling Trial Materials (may
Financial Agreement   ☐ be in protocol or Investigator's Brochure)   ☐
Insurance Statement/Indemnity   ☐ Records of Transportation of Trial Materials ☐
Other Signed Agreements   ☐ Code Break Procedure   ☐
Ethics Committee Approval ☐ Amendments ☐
Ethics Committee Composition   ☐

Trial Initiation Report   ☐ Details of Subjects Actively Screened   ⎫ may all   ☐
Correspondence   ☐ Names and Study Numbers of all Subjects ⎬ be one   ☐
Meeting Reports   ☐ Chronological List of Subjects Entered   ⎭ document   ☐
Telephone Call Notes   ☐ Drug Accountability Records   ☐
Source Documents   ☐ Specimen Signatures/Initials/Responsibilities   ☐
Copies of Completed CRFs   ☐ Record of retained samples   ☐
Copies of CRF Corrections (data query
   resolutions)   ☐
Serious Adverse Event Reports   ☐
Safety Reports to Regulatory Authorities ☐
Safety Updates from Sponsor (may be in
   correspondence)   ☐
Reports to Ethics Committee   ☐

Drug Destruction or Return Records   ☐ Notification to Ethics Committee of Completion   ☐
Trial Report (may be archived later)   ☐

SOP 26 – CHECKLIST
Archiving

Name of Principal Investigator _____ _____

                                                 (Forename)   *(Surname)*

Precise location/Address of archive _____

_____

_____

Archive for patient source documents, if different from above address:

Precise location/Address of archive _____

_____

_____

Date of earliest possible ⌷⌷   ⌷⌷   Sponsor to be notified of this date

destruction of archived   month   year   ☐ (✓ when done in writing)

documents:

Checklist completed by: _____ *on* _____

                                                                  (date)

SOP 27
Audits and Inspections

Background

In the three big pharma markets of Europe, USA and Japan, and increasingly in the other markets, the regulatory authorities demand that the Sponsor has a quality assurance system for submitted data to the registration authorities for registration approval. The authorities reserve the right to check the so-called source data, original data and patients' data with both the Sponsor and the Investigator. It may depend on the result of this inspection whether the registration will be allowed or denied. Generally speaking, there are two kinds of audit: that by a Sponsor or its agent, or an audit by a regulatory authority (which is often referred to as an inspection).

SOP 27
Audits and Inspections

Purpose

The purpose of this SOP is to describe the requirements for an audit or inspection of the study site.

Other Related Procedures

All SOPS. Auditors will probably audit against the SOPs in place at the site

Procedure

1. Who?

The following personnel, where appropriate, should be available to answer questions and for the final meeting before the auditor leaves the site:

- Principal Investigator
- Research Registrar
- Any doctor involved directly or indirectly during the study
- Study Site Co-ordinator/Research Nurse
- Trials Pharmacist
- Laboratory staff
- X-ray department staff
- Any person involved in performing tests during the study.

It may be that the auditor will request to visit certain departments. If so, colleagues should be told beforehand.

2. When?

Audits can take place prior to, during and after the patient recruitment phase, although the latter is uncommon unless it is an audit by a regulatory authority. They may be called upon as part of the development process of a particular compound, when sites are particularly high recruiters (the opposite is also true) or if there is any cause for concern, a 'for cause' audit.

Sufficient time should be given to those expected to attend the audit allowing them to plan their time around the day's activities.

3. How?

The following items may be audited and must be kept up to date:

a) Investigator Study File
b) Case record forms
c) Patient case notes
d) Pharmacy and drug records

SOP 27
Audits and Inspections

a) Investigator's Study File

The Investigator's Study File should be easy to follow and complete for audit. Prior to the audit ensure that the following items are present and up to date in the site Study File:

Trial Initiation Report
Monitoring visits log
Up-to-date Clinical Investigator's Brochure (and record of updates)
Confirmation of Regulatory Approval
Signed trial agreement (if this is separate from protocol and financial agreement)
Signed copy of the final protocol and any amendments
Specimen case record forms
Specimen diary card, questionnaires etc.
Dated, signed CVs of all study site personnel
Specimen of signatures of site staff
Responsibilities list
Signed FDA 1572 form (IND studies)
Correspondence and communication with the sponsoring company
Record relating to equipment loan during the study
Equipment calibration logs
Laboratory certification (including updates)
Laboratory normal reference ranges (including updates)
Standard letter to GP informing them the patient has entered the trial
Details of any CRF changes recorded on separate correction documents
Record of retained samples (blood etc.)

Details of the whereabouts of all archived study data should be available for the auditor and an assurance from the Principal Investigator that the data will be maintained according to the laws of GCP.

Finances
Signed financial agreement
Copies of receipts or financial correspondence

Pharmacy
Pharmacy agreement
Drug log and associated pharmacy documentation
Records of receipt and return (or destruction) of drug at site
All dispensing records
Randomisation codes

Drug handling details (if not in Investigator's Brochure)

SOP 27
Audits and Inspections

Ethics

Any correspondence with the Ethics Committee
List of Committee members
Letter of Ethics Committee approval and approval of any protocol amendments or other changes
Copy of Ethics Committee Application Form (completed)
Annual progress report to Committee
Notification of end of study
Insurance statement (where required, if not part of subject information sheet, protocol or other documentation)
Signed indemnity letter
Any advertisement for subject recruitment
Specimen subject information sheet
Specimen consent form (where separate)
Signed consent forms
Subject screening list
Subject recruitment log
Subject identification record
Copies of reports of serious adverse events

b) Case record forms

Ensure that:

All case record forms are available for the auditors
All CRFs are as complete as possible
All amendments are made correctly
Dates of patient visits match recruitment logs
Laboratory results, x-ray results etc. are present
All trials details are filed in the appropriate place.

c) Patient case notes

Ensure all patients' notes are available for checking. This should include all records, GP letters, laboratory results, x-ray results etc. from the trial. If any notes are not available provide the auditor with a reason.

SOP 27
Audits and Inspections

d) Pharmacy and drug records

Pharmacy and drug records should be checked in advance to ensure that:

Dispensing dates match up with visit dates
Drug logs are complete
Tablet counts are recorded
All drug returns are counted
Boxes containing drugs for return are labelled for return
Drug storage is appropriately recorded
Drug dispensing is appropriately recorded
Pharmacy has copies of correspondence with Sponsor, including a financial agreement, protocol and written dispensing details, plus Investigator's Brochure where appropriate.

SOP approved by: _____

Signature: _____ *Date:* _____

SOP 27 – CHECKLIST
Audits and Inspections

Protocol Code: [_____]   Date of Protocol: [_|_|_|_]
dd mm yy

Abbreviated Title: _____

Sponsor Name: _____

	Details
On which date(s) has the audit been agreed for?	
Is there correspondence between the site and the Monitor detailing the audit/inspection plans, date and time?	
Will an interpreter be required? If yes, what arrangements have been made?	
Review the protocol and give details of any known deviations with reasons.	
Review the Standard Operating Procedures and note details of any omissions or deviations, with reasons.	
Check the Study File for presence of all signed documents. Note any that are missing and action taken.	
Are any other documents known to be missing from the study master file?	
Where will the auditor be able to work (in peace, with space to layout documents)?	
Enter the study subjects' numbers for which case record forms are available for audit. This should be for all CRFs.	
If original medical records are not available for all subjects, record details and reasons.	
Have all subjects consented to their medical records being viewed? If not, give details and details of how any review of notes will be managed.	
Which site personnel will be available? Give details of times (and dates). Has this been agreed with the auditor?	
What arrangements are there in the event the auditor needs to make copies of documents?	

Checklist completed by: _____ *on* _____

(date)

FDA Regulations Concerning Clinical Trials

This is a summary of the FDA Regulations affecting clinical trials, concentrating on the procedure and requirements for informed consent, Ethics Committee approval (Ethics Committees are called Institutional Review Boards (IRB) in the FDA legislation), responsibilities of the Investigator and documentation, record keeping and record retention. Although the USA has adopted the ICH Harmonized Tripartite Guidelines for Good Clinical Practice, the FDA Regulations are also still accepted. This section is included in case you are asked to comply with the FDA Regulations.

FDA Regulations – Informed Consent

The FDA Regulations for informed consent are more detailed than either the old European or the ICH Guidelines. In studies performed in Europe for the FDA, informed consent is one of the main areas where there are problems because of non-compliance with the FDA Regulations.

All guidelines require the study to comply with the principles of informed consent as outlined in the Declaration of Helsinki; the USA requires written consent, the ICH may be written or oral. If a European study is being conducted under Investigational New Drug regulations, and written consent as defined by the FDA guidelines is not being obtained, then it is important that the FDA be informed and a waiver be obtained in writing from the FDA.

No Investigator may involve a patient in a clinical study without first obtaining from the patient an informed consent.

The patient must be given sufficient opportunity to decide whether to participate, without undue pressure or influence from the Investigator.

In seeking informed consent, the following information shall be provided to each subject:

1. A statement that the study involves research, an explanation of the purposes of the research, the expected duration of the subject's participation, a description of the procedures to be followed and identification of any procedures which are experimental.
2. A description of any reasonably foreseeable risks or discomfort to the subject.
3. A description of any benefits to the subject or to others which may reasonably be expected from the research.
4. A disclosure of appropriate alternative procedures or courses of treatment, if any, that might be advantageous to the subject.
5. A statement regarding the extent, if any, to which confidentiality of records identifying the subject will be maintained and that notes the possibility that the FDA may inspect the records.
6. For research involving more than minimal risk, an explanation as to whether any compensation and an explanation as to whether any medical treatments are available if injury occurs and, if so, what they consist of, or whether further information may be obtained.

7. An explanation of whom to contact for answers to pertinent questions about the research and research subject's rights, and whom to contact in the event of a research-related injury to the subject.
8. A statement that participation is voluntary, that refusal to participate will involve no penalty or loss of benefits to which the subject is otherwise entitled, and that the subject may discontinue participation at any time without penalty or loss of benefits to which the subject is otherwise entitled.

Additional Elements of Informed Consent

When appropriate, one or more of the following elements of information shall also be provided for the subject:

1. A statement that the particular treatment or procedure may involve risks to the subject (or to the embryo or foetus, if the subject is or may become pregnant) which are currently unforeseeable.
2. Anticipated circumstances under which the subject's participation may be terminated by the Investigator without regard to the subject's consent.
3. Any additional costs to the subject that may result from participation in the research.
4. The consequences of a subject's decision to withdraw from the research and procedures for orderly termination of participation by the subject.
5. A statement that significant new findings developed during the course of the research which may relate to the subject's willingness to continue participation will be provided to the subject.
6. The approximate number of subjects involved in the study.

The informed consent requirements in these regulations are not intended to prompt any applicable federal, state or local laws which require additional information to be disclosed for informed consent to be legally effective.

Nothing in these regulations is intended to limit the authority of a physician to provide emergency medical care to the extent the physician is permitted to do so under applicable federal, state or local law.

Possible Problems with Informed Consent

Informed consent may be considered as being inadequate if it concentrates more on benefits than on discomfort which may be caused by the trial, or by revealing to a subject too blatantly the inevitable nature of his or her disorder. The manner in which consent was obtained may be suspect because of pressure exerted on subjects. There are often difficulties in assessing the adequacy of the informed consent because of different medical and cultural habits, particularly differences between American and European behaviour.

Documentation of Informed Consent

Informed consent shall be documented by the use of a written consent form approved by the IRB and signed by the subject or the subject's legally authorised representative. A copy shall be given to the person signing the form.

The consent form may be either of the following:

- A written consent document that embodies the elements of informed consent listed above. This form may be read to the subject or the subject's legally authorised representative, but, in any event, the Investigator shall give either the subject or the representative adequate opportunity to read it before it is signed.
- A 'short form' written consent document stating that the elements of informed consent required have been presented orally to the subject or the subject's legally authorised representative. When this method is used, there shall be a witness to the oral presentation. Also, the IRB shall approve a written summary of what is to be said to the subject or the representative. Only the short form itself is to be signed by the subject or the representative. However, the witness shall sign both the short form and a copy of the summary, and the person actually obtaining the consent shall sign a copy of the summary. A copy of the summary shall be given to the subject or the representative in addition to a copy of the short form.

FDA Regulations – Institutional Review Boards

Organisation and Personnel

Institutional Review Board means any board, committee or other group formally designated by an institution to review, to approve the initiation of, and to conduct periodic review of, biomedical research involving human subjects. The primary purpose of such review is to assure the protection of the rights and welfare of human subjects.

IRB Membership

Each IRB shall have at least five members, with varying backgrounds, to promote complete and adequate review of research activities commonly conducted by the institution. The IRB shall be sufficiently qualified through the experience and expertise of its members, and the diversity of the members' backgrounds, including consideration of the racial and cultural backgrounds of members and sensitivity to such issues as community attitudes, to promote respect for its advice and counsel in safeguarding the rights and welfare of human subjects. In addition to possessing the professional competence necessary to review specific research activities, the IRB shall be able to ascertain the acceptability of proposed research in terms of institutional commitments and regulations, applicable law, and standards of professional conduct and practice. The IRB shall therefore include persons knowledgeable in these areas. If an IRB regularly reviews research that involves a vulnerable category of subjects, including but not limited to subjects covered by other parts of this chapter, the IRB should include one or more individuals who are primarily concerned with the welfare of these subjects.

No IRB may consist entirely of men, or entirely of women, or entirely of members of one profession.

Each IRB shall include at least one member whose primary concerns are in non-scientific areas; for example: lawyers, ethicists, members of the clergy.

Each IRB shall include at least one member who is not otherwise affiliated with the institution and who is not part of the immediate family of a person who is affiliated with the institution.

No IRB may have a member participate in the IRB's initial or continuing review of any project in which the member has a conflicting interest, except to provide information requested by the IRB.

An IRB may, in its discretion, invite individuals with competence in special areas to assist in the review of complex issues which require expertise beyond or in addition to that available on the IRB. These individuals may not vote with the IRB.

IRB Functions and Operations

The exact functions and operations of the IRB are listed in the FDA Regulations, including the ethical criteria which should be examined for each study. The IRB must maintain adequate documentation of its activities, including minutes of meetings, copies of correspondence, copies of submitted documents, and a list of members of the IRB. This documentation must be available for inspection by the FDA.

FDA Investigator Responsibilities

Definition of an Investigator

'Investigator' means an individual who actually conducts a clinical investigation (i.e. under whose immediate direction the drug is administered to a subject).

If an investigation is conducted by a team of individuals, the Investigator is the responsible leader of the team. 'Sub-Investigator' includes any other individual member of that team.

Only Investigators qualified by training and experience may participate in clinical trials, and only these Investigators may receive supplies of the investigational new drug.

Duties of the Investigator – Form FDA 1572

Sponsored clinical research studies are subject to the regulations of the US Food and Drug Administration (FDA). The responsibilities imposed upon Investigators by the FDA are summarised in the 'Statement of Investigator' (Form FDA 1572), which is actually a form letter addressed to the Sponsor summarising the Investigator's qualifications for the study and his or her willingness to follow FDA Regulations with respect to the study.

Each Investigator must complete and sign Form FDA 1572. The following information must be provided on the form:

- A CV or other statement of qualifications must be attached to the form to verify that the Investigator is an expert in the clinical investigation of the drug for the use under investigation.

- Names and addresses of the Investigator, facility where the investigation is to be conducted, clinical laboratory facilities, IRB and the names of the Sub-Investigators must all be listed, along with the name and code number of the protocol.

Clinical Protocol Information must also be attached – this will depend on the phase of the study. For Phase III studies it must include:

- An outline of the study protocol including an approximation of the number of subjects to be treated with the drug and number to be employed as controls, if any.
- The clinical uses to be investigated.
- Characteristics of subjects by age, sex and condition.
- The kind of clinical observations and laboratory tests to be conducted.
- The estimated duration of the study.
- Copies or descriptions of the case report forms being used.

In signing the form the Investigator agrees to:

- Conduct the study in accordance with the relevant, current protocol and only make changes in a protocol after notifying the Sponsor, except when necessary to protect the safety, the rights or welfare of subjects.
- Comply with all requirements regarding the obligations of clinical Investigators and all other pertinent requirements in this part.
- Personally conduct or supervise the described investigations.
- Inform any patients, or any persons used as controls, that the drugs are being used for investigational purposes and ensure that the requirements relating to obtaining informed consent and IRB review and approval are met.
- Report to the Sponsor adverse experiences that occur in the course of the investigations.
- Maintain adequate and accurate records in accordance with the FDA Regulations and make those records available for inspection.
- Read and understand the information in the Investigator's Brochure, including the potential risks and side effects of the drug.
- Ensure that all associates, colleagues and employees assisting in the conduct of the study are informed about their obligations in meeting the above commitments.
- Ensure that the IRB conforms to FDA Regulations and will be responsible for the initial and continuing review and approval of the clinical investigation. The Investigator agrees to promptly report to the IRB all changes in the research activity and all unanticipated problems involving risks to human subjects or others. The Investigator will not make any changes in the research without IRB approval, except where necessary to eliminate apparent immediate hazards to human subjects.

Documentation, Record Keeping and Record Retention

The Sponsor has the obligation to ensure that the study will be conducted by qualified Investigators with sufficient resources (of time, personnel and physical facilities) to conduct the study and to ensure that the Investigator understands and agrees to comply with applicable regulations, policies and procedures. Prior to the beginning of any clinical study, each Investigator will be asked to provide the following documentation:

1. A signed protocol for the study.
2. A signed form FDA 1572 certifying the Investigator's agreement to comply with US regulations governing the conduct of the study.
3. A CV of the Investigator. If Sub-Investigators will participate in the study, a CV for each.
4. A copy of the letter of approval of the Institutional Review Board (IRB).
5. A list of members of the IRB, including their occupations and institutional affiliations.
6. A specimen copy of the IRB-approved informed consent document to be used in the study, clearly indicating the date of IRB approval.
7. A list of normal ranges of values for all local laboratory tests specified by the protocol and all laboratories utilised.
8. A copy of the local laboratory(ies) certification(s) or the number of the certification(s), the name of the certifying authority, and the period of certification.

Investigator Record Keeping and Record Retention

1. Disposition of drug

An Investigator is required to maintain adequate records of the disposition of the drug, including dates, quantity and use by subjects. If the investigation is terminated, suspended, discontinued or completed, the Investigator shall return the unused supplies of the drug to the Sponsor, or dispose of the drug as arranged with the Sponsor.

2. Case histories

An Investigator is required to prepare and maintain adequate case histories designed to record all observations and other data pertinent to the investigation on each individual treated with the investigational drug or employed as a control in the investigation.

3. Record retention

An Investigator shall retain records for a minimum period of two years following application approval of the indication, or for two years after the investigation is discontinued and the FDA is notified.

Index

Index compiled by Anne McCarthy